A Clinician's Guide to Statistics and Epidemiology in Mental Health

A Clinician's Guide to Statistics and Epidemiology in Mental Health

Measuring Truth and Uncertainty

S. Nassir Ghaemi MD MPH

Professor of Psychiatry, Tufts University School of Medicine
Director, Mood Disorders Program, Tufts Medical Center
Boston, Massachusetts

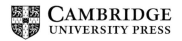
CAMBRIDGE
UNIVERSITY PRESS

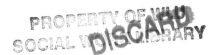

CAMBRIDGE UNIVERSITY PRESS
Cambridge, New York, Melbourne, Madrid, Cape Town, Singapore,
São Paulo, Delhi

Cambridge University Press
The Edinburgh Building, Cambridge CB2 8RU, UK

Published in the United States of America
by Cambridge University Press, New York

www.cambridge.org
Information on this title:
www.cambridge.org/9780521709583

First published 2009

Printed in the United Kingdom at the University Press, Cambridge

*A catalog record for this publication is available from the British
Library*

Library of Congress Cataloging in Publication data
Ghaemi, S. Nassir.
A clinician's guide to statistics and epidemiology in mental health :
measuring truth and uncertainty / S. Nassir Ghaemi.
    p. ; cm.
Includes bibliographical references and index.
ISBN 978-0-521-70958-3 (pbk.)
1. Psychiatry – Statistical methods.   2. Psychiatric epidemiology.
I. Title.
[DNLM: 1. Psychiatry – methods.   2. Statistics as Topic.
3. Mental Disorders – epidemiology.   WM 30 G411c   2009]
RC467.8.G53   2009
362.2′0422 – dc22   2009019273

ISBN 978-0-521-70958-3 paperback

To my father, Kamal Ghaemi MD
and my mother, Guity Kamali Ghaemi

Errors in judgment must occur in the practice of an art which consists largely of balancing probabilities.

William Osler (Osler, 1932; p. 38)

The genius of statistics, as Laplace defined it, was that it did not ignore errors; it quantified them.

(Menand, 2001; p. 182)

Contents

Preface

Medicine without statistics is quackery; statistics without medicine is numerology. Perhaps this is the main reason why clinicians should care about statistics.

Statistics in medicine began in the early nineteenth century (it was called "the numerical method" then) and its debut involved disproving the most common and widely accepted medical treatment for millennia: bleeding. From ancient Rome until 1900, all physicians – from Galen to Avicenna to Benjamin Rush – strongly and clearly advocated bleeding as the treatment for most medical illnesses. This was based on a theory, most clearly defined by Galen: four humors in the body, if out of balance, led to disease; bleeding rebalanced the humors.

Of course this was all wrong. Even the dullest physician today would know better. How was it disproven?

Statistics.

Pierre Louis, the founder of the numerical method, counted 40 patients with pneumonia treated with bleeding and showed that the more they were treated, the sooner they died. Bleeding did not treat pneumonia, it worsened it (Louis, 1835).

Counting – that was the essence of the numerical method; and it remains the essence of statistics. If you can count, you can understand statistics. And if you can't (or won't) count, you should not treat patients.

Simply counting patients showed that the vaunted experience of the great medical geniuses of the past was all for nought. And if Galen and Avicenna could be mistaken, so can you.

The essence of the need for medical statistics is that you cannot count on your own experience, you cannot believe your eyes, you cannot simply practice medicine based on what you think you observe. If you do this, you are practicing pre-nineteenth century, prescientific, prestatistical medicine.

The bleeding of today, in other words, could well be the Prozac or the psychotherapy that so many of us mental health clinicians prescribe. We should not do things just because everyone else is doing it, or because our teachers told us so. In medicine, the life and death of our patients hang in the balance; we need better reasons for preserving life, or causing death, than simply opinion: we need facts, science ... statistics.

Clinicians need statistics, then, to practice scientifically and ethically. The problem is that many, if not most, doctors and clinicians, though trained in biology and anatomy, fear numbers; mathematics is foreign to them, statistics alien.

There is no way around it though; without counting, medicine is not scientific. So how can we get around this fear and begin to teach statistics to clinicians?

I find that clinicians whom I meet in the course of lectures, primarily about psychopharmacology, crave this kind of framing of how to read and analyze research studies. Residents and students also are rarely and only minimally exposed to such ideas in training, and, in the course of journal club experiences, I find that they clearly benefit from a systematic exposition of how to assess evidence. Many of the confusing interpretations heard by clinicians are due to their own inability to critically read the literature. They are aware of this fact, but are unable to understand standard statistical texts. They need a book that simply describes what they need to know and is directly relevant to their clinical interests. I have not found such a book that I could recommend to them.

So I decided to write it.

A final preliminary comment, aimed more at statisticians than clinicians. This book does not seek to teach you how to *do* statistics (though the Appendix provides some instruction on conducting regression analysis); it seeks to teach you how to *understand* statistics. It is for the clinician or researcher who wants to understand what he or she is doing or seeing; not for a statistician who wants to run a specific test. There are no discussions of parametric versus non-parametric tests here; plenty of textbooks written by statisticians exist for that purpose. This is a book *by* a clinical researcher in psychiatry *for* clinicians and researchers in the mental health professions. It is not written for statisticians, many of whom will, I expect, find it unsatisfying. Matters of professional territoriality are hard to avoid. I suppose I might feel the same if a statistician tried to write a book about bipolar disorder. I am sure I have certain facts wrong, and that some misinterpretations of detail exist. But it cannot be helped, when one deals with matters that are interdisciplinary; some discipline or another will feel out of sorts. I believe, however, that the large conceptual structure of the book is sound, and that most of its ideas are reasonably defensible. So, I hope statisticians do not look at this book, see it as superficial or incomplete, and then simply dismiss it. They are not the ones who need to read it. And I hope that clinicians will take a look, despite their aversion to statistics, and realize that this was written for them.

Acknowledgements

This book reflects how I have integrated what I learned in the course of Master of Public Health (MPH) coursework in the Clinical Effectiveness Program at the Harvard School of Public Health. Before I entered that program in 2002, I had been a psychiatric researcher for almost a decade. When I left that program in 2004, I was completely changed. I had gone into the program thinking I would gain technical knowledge that would help me manipulate numbers; and I did. But more importantly, I learned how to understand, conceptually, what the numbers meant. I became a much better researcher, and a better teacher, and a better peer reviewer, I think. I look back on my pre-MPH days as an era of amateur research almost. My two main teachers in the Clinical Effectiveness Program, guides for hundreds of researchers that have gone through their doors for decades, were the epidemiologist Francis Cook and the statistician John Orav. Of course they cannot be held responsible for any specific content in this book, which reflects my own, sometimes contrarian, and certainly at times mistaken, views. Where I am wrong, I take full responsibility; where correct, they deserve the credit for putting me on a new and previously unknown path. Of them Emerson's words hold true: a teacher never knows where his influence ends; it can stretch on to eternity.

I would not have been able to take that MPH course of study without the support of a Research Career Development Award (K-23 grant: MH-64189) from the National Institute of Mental Health. Those awards are designed for young researchers, and include a teaching component which is meant to advance the formal research skills of the recipient. This concept certainly applied well to me, and I hope that this book can be seen in part as the product of taxpayer funds well spent.

Through many lectures, I expressed my enthusiasm to share my new insights about research and statistics, a process of give and take with experienced and intelligent clinicians which led to this book. My friend Jacob Katzow, perhaps the longest continual psychopharmacologist in clinical practice in Washington DC, consistently encouraged me to seek to bridge this clinician/researcher divide and helped me to keep talking the language of clinicians, even when describing the concepts of statisticians. Federico Soldani, who worked with me as a research fellow before pursuing a PhD in public health at Harvard, helped me greatly in our constant discussion and study of research methodologies in psychiatry. Frederick K. Goodwin, always a mentor to me, also has continually encouraged this part of my academic work, as has Ross Baldessarini. With a secondary appointment on the faculty of the Emory School of Public Health in recent years, I made the friendship of Howard Kushner, who also helped mature some of my epidemiological and public health-oriented thinking. Among psychiatric colleagues who share my passion on this topic, Franco Benazzi read an early draft, and Eric Smith provided important comments that I incorporated in Chapters 4–6. Richard Marley at Cambridge University Press first suggested this project to me, persisted in his request even after I expressed reservations, tolerated my passive-aggressive tardiness in the face of a daunting task, and, in the end, accepted the only end result I could produce, not a straightforward text, but a critique. Not all editors and publishers would be so patient and flexible.

My family continues to tolerate the unique gift, and danger, of the life of the academic: even when at home, ideas still roam around in one's mind, and there is no end to the potential effort of reading and writing. They set the limits, and provide the rewards, that I need.

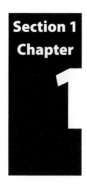

Section 1
Chapter

1

Basic concepts
Why data never speak
for themselves

Science teaches us to doubt, and in ignorance, to refrain.

Claude Bernard (Silverman, 1998; p. 1)

The beginning of wisdom is to recognize our own ignorance. We mental health clinicians need to start by acknowledging that we are ignorant; we do not know what to do; if we did, we would not need to read anything, much less this book – we could then just treat our patients with the infallible knowledge that we already possess. Although there are dogmatists (and many of them) of this variety – who think that they can be good mental health professionals by simply applying the truths of, say, Freud (or Prozac) to all – this book is addressed to those who know that they do not know, or who at least want to know more.

When faced with persons with mental illnesses, we clinicians need to first determine what their problems are, and then what kinds of treatments to give them. In both cases, in particular the matter of treatment, we need to turn somewhere for guidance: how should we treat patients?

We no longer live in the era of Galen: pointing to the opinions of a wise man is insufficient (though many still do this). Many have accepted that we should turn to science; some kind of empirical research should guide us.

If we accept this view – that science is our guide – then the first question is how are we to understand science?

Science is not simple

This book would be unnecessary if science was simple. I would like to disabuse the reader of any simple notion of science, specifically "positivism": the view that science consists of positive facts, piled on each other one after another, each of which represents an absolute truth, or an independent reality, our business being simply to discover those truths or realities.

This is simply not the case. Science is much more complex.

For the past century scientists and philosophers have debated this matter, and it comes down to this: facts cannot be separated from theories; science involves deduction, and not just induction. In this way, no facts are observed without a preceding hypothesis. Sometimes, the hypothesis is not even fully formulated or even conscious; I may have a number of assumptions that direct me to look at certain facts. It is in this sense that philosophers say that facts are "theory-laden"; between fact and theory no sharp line can be drawn.

How statistics came to be

A broad outline of how statistics came to be is as follows (Salsburg, 2001): Statistics were developed in the eighteenth century because scientists and mathematicians began to recognize the inherent role of uncertainty in all scientific work. In physics and astronomy, for instance, Pierre Laplace realized that certain error was inherent in all calculations. Instead of ignoring the error, he chose to quantify it, and the field of statistics was born. He even showed that there was a mathematical distribution to the likelihood of errors observed in given experiments. Statistical notions were first explicitly applied to human beings by the nineteenth-century Belgian Lambert Adolphe Quetelet, who applied it to the normal population, and the nineteenth-century French physician Pierre Louis, who applied it to sick persons. In the late nineteenth-century, Francis Galton, a founder of genetics and a mathematical leader, applied it to human psychology (studies of intelligence) and worked out the probabilistic nature of statistical inference more fully. His student, Karl Pearson, then took Laplace one step further and showed that not only is there a probability to the likelihood of error, but even our own measurements are probabilities: "Looking at the data accumulated in biology, Pearson conceived the measurements themselves, rather than errors in the measurement, as having a probability distribution." (Salsburg, 2001; p. 16.) Pearson called our observed measurements "parameters" (Greek for "almost measurements"), and he developed staple notions like the mean and standard deviation. Pearson's revolutionary work laid the basis for modern statistics. But if he was the Marx of statistics (he actually was a socialist), the Lenin of statistics would be the early twentieth-century geneticist Ronald Fisher, who introduced randomization and p-values, followed by A. Bradford Hill in the mid twentieth-century, who applied these concepts to medical illnesses and founded clinical epidemiology. (The reader will see some of these names repeatedly in the rest of this book; the ideas of these thinkers form the basis of understanding statistics.)

It was Fisher who first coined the term "statistic" (Louis had called it the "numerical method"), by which he meant the observed measurements in an experiment, seen as a reflection of all possible measurements. It is "a number that is derived from the observed measurements and that estimates a parameter of the distribution." (Salsburg, 2001; p. 89.) He saw the observed measurement as a random number among the possible measurements that could have been made, and thus "since a statistic is random, it makes no sense to talk about how accurate a single value of it is … What is needed is a criterion that depends on the probability distribution of the statistic …" (Salsburg, 2001; p. 66). How probably valid is the observed measurement, asked Fisher? Statistical tests are all about establishing these probabilities, and statistical concepts are about how we can use mathematical probability to know whether our observations are more or less likely to be correct.

A scientific revolution

This process was really a revolution; it was a major change in our thinking about science. Prior to these developments, even the most enlightened thinkers (such as the French Encylopedists of the eighteenth century, and Auguste Comte in the nineteenth century) saw science as the process of developing absolutely certain knowledge through refinements of sense-observation. Statistics rests on the concept that scientific knowledge, derived from observation using our five senses aided by technologies, is not absolute. Hence, "the basic idea behind the statistical revolution is that the real things of science are distributions of number, which can then be described by parameters. It is mathematically convenient to embed that concept into probability theory and deal with probability distributions." (Salsburg, 2001; pp. 307–8.)

It is thus not an option to avoid statistics, if one cares about science. And if one understands science correctly, not as a matter of absolute positive knowledge but as a much more complex probabilistic endeavor (see Chapter 11), then statistics are part and parcel of science.

Some doctors hate statistics; but they claim to support science. They cannot have it both ways.

A benefit to humankind

Statistics thus developed outside of medicine, in other sciences in which researchers realized that uncertainty and error were in the nature of science. Once the wish for absolute truth was jettisoned, statistics would become an essential aspect of all science. And if physics involves uncertainty, how much more uncertainty is there in medicine? Human beings are much more uncertain than atoms and electrons.

The practical results of statistics in medicine are undeniable. If nothing else had been achieved but two things – in the nineteenth century, the end of bleeding, purging, and leeching as a result of Louis' studies (Louis, 1835); and in the twentieth century the proof of cigarette smoking related lung cancer as a result of Hill's studies (Hill, 1971) – we would have to admit that medical statistics have delivered humanity from two powerful scourges.

Numbers do not stand alone

The history of science shows us that scientific knowledge is not absolute, and that all science involves uncertainty. These truths lead us to a need for statistics. Thus, in learning about statistics, the reader should not expect pure facts; the result of statistical analyses is not unadorned and irrefutable fact; all statistics is an act of interpretation, and the result of statistics is more interpretation. This is, in reality, the nature of all science: it is all interpretation of facts, not simply facts by themselves.

This statistical reality – the fact that data do not speak for themselves and that therefore positivistic reliance on facts is wrong – is called *confounding bias*. As discussed in Chapter 2, observation is fallible: we sometimes think we see what is *not* in fact there. This is especially the case in research on human beings. Consider: caffeine causes cancer; numerous studies have shown this; the observation has been made over and over again: among those with cancer, coffee use is high compared to those without cancer. Those are the unadorned facts – and they are wrong. Why? Because coffee drinkers also smoke cigarettes more than non-coffee drinkers. Cigarettes are a confounding factor in this observation, and our lives are chock full of such confounding factors. Meaning: we cannot believe our eyes. Observation is not enough for science; one must try to observe *accurately*, by removing confounding factors. How? In two ways: 1. Experiment, by which we control all other factors in the environment except one, thus knowing that any changes are due to the impact of that one factor. This can be done with animals in a laboratory, but human beings cannot be controlled in this way (ethically). Enter the randomized clinical trial (RCT). These are how we experiment with humans to be able to observe accurately. 2. Statistics: certain methods (such as regression modeling, see Chapter 6) have been devised to mathematically correct for the impact of measured confounding factors.

We thus need statistics, either through the design of RCTs or through special analyses, so that we can make our observations accurate, and so that we can correctly (and not spuriously) accept or reject our hypotheses.

Science is about hypotheses and hypothesis-testing, about confirmation and refutation, about confounding bias and experiment, about RCTs and statistical analysis: in a word, it is not just about facts. Facts always need to be interpreted. And that is the job of statistics: not to tell us the truth, but to help us get closer to the truth by understanding how to interpret the facts.

Knowing less, doing more

That is the goal of this book. If you are a researcher, perhaps this book will explain why you do some of the things you do in your analyses and studies, and how you might improve them. If you are a clinician, hopefully it will put you in a place where you can begin to make independent judgments about studies, and not simply be at the mercy of the interpretations of others. It may help you realize that the facts are much more complex than they seem; you may end up "knowing" less than you do now, in the sense that you will realize that much that passes for knowledge is only one among other interpretations, but at the same time I hope this statistical wisdom proves liberating: you will be less at the mercy of numbers and more in charge of knowing how to interpret numbers. You will know less, but at the same time, what you do know will be more valid and more solid, and thus you will become a better clinician: applying accurate knowledge rather than speculation, and being more clearly aware of where the region of our knowledge ends and where the realm of our ignorance begins.

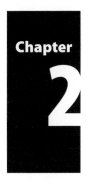

Chapter

2 Why you cannot believe your eyes: the Three C's

Believe nothing you hear, and only one half that you see.

Edgar Allan Poe (Poe, 1845)

A core concept in this book is that the validity of any study involves the sequential assessment of Confounding bias, followed by Chance, followed by Causation (what has been called the Three C's) (Abramson and Abramson, 2001).

Any study needs to pass these three hurdles before you should consider accepting its results. Once we accept that no fact or study result is accepted at face value (because no facts can be observed purely, but rather all are interpreted), then we can turn to statistics to see what kinds of methods we should use to analyze those facts. These three steps are widely accepted and form the core of statistics and epidemiology.

The first C: bias (confounding)

The first step is bias, by which we mean *systematic* error (as opposed to the random error of chance). Systematic error means that one makes the same mistake over and over again because of some inherent problem with the observations being made. There are subtypes of bias (selection, confounding, measurement), and they are all important, but I will emphasize here what is perhaps the most common and insufficiently appreciated kind of bias: confounding. Confounding has to do with factors, of which we are unaware, that influence our observed results. The concept is best visualized in Figure 2.1.

Hormone replacement therapy

As seen in Figure 2.1, the confounding factor is associated with the exposure (or what we think is the cause) and leads to the result. The *real* cause is the confounding factor; the *apparent* cause, which we observe, is just along for the ride. The example of caffeine, cigarettes, and cancer was given in Chapter 1. Another key example is the case of hormone replacement therapy (HRT). For decades, with much observational experience and large observational studies, most physicians were convinced that HRT had beneficial medical effects in women, especially postmenopausally. Those women who used HRT did better than those who did not use HRT. When finally put to the test in a huge randomized clinical trial (RCT), HRT was found to lead to actually worse cardiovascular and cancer outcomes than placebo. Why had the observational results been wrong? Because of confounding bias: those women who had used HRT also had better diets and exercised more than women who did not use HRT. Diet and exercise were the confounding factors: they led to better medical outcomes directly, and they were associated with HRT. When the RCT equalized all women who received HRT versus placebo on diet and exercise (as well as all other factors), the direct effect of HRT could

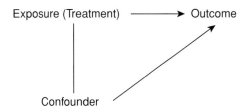

Figure 2.1 Confounding bias.

finally be observed accurately; and it was harmful to boot (Prentice *et al.*, 2006). (This example is discussed more in Chapter 9.)

The eternal triangle

As one author puts it: "Confounding is the epidemiologist's eternal triangle. Any time a risk factor, patient characteristic, or intervention appears to be causing a disease, side effect, or outcome, the relationship needs to be challenged. Are we seeing cause and effect, or is a confounding factor exerting its unappreciated influence? ... Confounding factors are always lurking, ready to cast doubt on the interpretation of studies." (Gehlbach, 2006; pp. 227–8.)

This is the lesson of confounding bias: *we cannot believe our eyes.* Or perhaps more accurately, we cannot be sure when our observations are right, and when they are wrong. Sometimes they are one way or the other, but, more often than not, observation is wrong rather than right due to the high prevalence of confounding factors in the world of medical care.

The kind of confounding bias that led to the HRT debacle had to do with intrinsic characteristics of the population. The doctors had nothing to do with the patients' diets and exercise; the patients themselves controlled those factors. It could turn out that completely independent features, such as hair color or age or gender, are confounding factors in any particular study. These are not controlled by patients or doctors; they are just there in the population and they can affect the results. Two other types of confounding factors exist which are the result of the behavior of patients and doctors: confounding by indication, and measurement bias.

Confounding by indication

The major confounding factor that results from the behavior of doctors is *confounding by indication* (also called selection bias). This is a classic and extremely poorly appreciated source of confusion in medical research:

As a clinician, you are trained to be a non-randomized treater. What this means is that you are taught, through years of supervision and more years of clinical experience, to tailor your treatment decisions to each individual patient. You do not treat patients randomly. You do not say to patient A, take drug X; and to patient B, take drug Y; and to patient C, take drug X; and to patient D, take drug Y – you do not do this without thinking any further about the matter, about why each patient should receive the one drug and not the other. You do not practice randomly; if you did, you should be appropriately sued. However, by practicing non-randomly, you automatically bias all your experience. You think your patients are doing well because of your treatments, whereas they should be doing well because you are tailoring your treatments *to those who would do well with them.* In other words, it often is not the treatment effects that you are observing, but the treatment effects in specially chosen populations. If you then generalize from those specific patients to the wider population of patients, you will be mistaken.

Measurement bias: blinding

I have focused on the first C as confounding bias. The larger topic here is bias, or systematic error, and besides confounding bias, there is one other major source of bias: measurement bias (sometimes also called information bias). Here the issue is not that the outcomes are due to unanalyzed confounding factors, but rather that the outcomes themselves may be inaccurate. The way the outcomes are measured, or the information on which the outcomes are based, is false. Often this can be related to the impact of either the patients' wishes or the doctors' beliefs; thus double-blinding is the usual means of handling measurement bias.

Randomization is the best means of addressing confounding bias, and blinding the means for measurement bias. While blinding is important, it is not as important as randomization. Confounding bias is much more prominent and multivaried than measurement bias. Clinicians often focus on blinding as the means of handling bias; this only addresses the minor part of bias. Unless randomization occurs, or regression modeling or other statistical analyses are conducted, the problem of confounding bias will render study results invalid.

The second C: chance

If a study is randomized and blinded successfully, or if observational data are appropriately analyzed with regression or other methods, and there still seems to be a relationship between a treatment and an outcome, we can then turn to the question of chance. We can then say that this relationship does not seem to be systematically erroneous due to some hidden bias in our observations; now the question is whether it just happened by chance, whether it represents *random* error.

I will discuss the nature of the hypothesis-testing approach in statistics in more detail in Chapter 8; suffice it to say here that the convention is that a relationship is viewed as being unlikely erroneous due to chance if, using mathematical equations designed to measure chance occurrence of associations, it is likely to have occurred 5% of the time, or less frequently, due to chance. This is the famous p-value, which I will discuss more in Chapter 7.

The application of those mathematical equations is a simple matter, and thus the assessment of chance is not complex at all. It is much simpler than assessing bias, but it is correspondingly less important. Usually, it is no big deal to assess chance; bias is the tough part. Yet again many clinicians equate statistics with p-values and assessing chance. This is one of the least important parts of statistics.

Often what happens is that the first C is ignored, bias is insufficiently examined, and the second C is exaggerated: not just 1, or 2, but 20 or 50 p-values are thrust upon the reader in the course of an article. The p-value is abused until it becomes useless, or, worse, misleading (see Chapter 7).

The problem with chance, usually, is that we focus too much on it, and we misinterpret our statistics. The problem with bias, usually, is we focus too little on it, and we don't even bother with statistics to assess it.

The third C: causation

Should a study pass the first two hurdles, bias and chance, it still should not be seen as valid unless we assess it in terms of causation. This is an even more complex topic, and a part of statistics where clinicians cannot simply look for a number or a p-value to give them an answer. We actually have to use our minds here, and think in terms of ideas, and not simply numbers.

The problem of causation is this: if X is associated with Y, and there is no bias or chance error, still we need to then show that X causes Y. Not just that Prozac *is associated with* less depression, but that Prozac *causes* less depression. How can we do this? A p-value will not do it for us.

This is a problem that has been central to the field of clinical epidemiology for decades. The classic handling of it has been ascribed to the work of the great medical epidemiologist A. Bradford Hill, who was central to the research on tobacco and lung cancer. A major problem with that research was that randomized studies could not be done: you smoke, you don't, and see me in 40 years to see who has cancer. This could not practically or ethically be done. This research was observational and liable to bias; Hill and others devised methods to assess bias, but they always had the problem of never being able to remove doubt completely. The cigarette companies, of course, constantly exploited this matter to magnify this doubt and delay the inevitable day when they would be forced to back off on their dangerous business.

With all this observational research, they would argue to Hill and his colleagues, you still cannot prove that cigarettes *cause* lung cancer. And they were right. So Hill set about trying to clarify how one might prove that something causes anything in medical research with human beings.

I will discuss this topic in more detail in Chapter 10. Hill basically pointed out that causation cannot be derived from any one source, but that it could be inferred by an accumulation of evidence from multiple sources (see Table 10.1).

It is not enough to say a study is valid; one also wants to know if these results are replicated by multiple studies, if they are supported by biological studies in animals on mechanisms of effect, if they follow certain patterns consistent with causation (like a dose–response relationship) and so on.

For our purposes, we might at least insist on replication. No single study should stand on its own, no matter how well done. Even after crossing the barriers of bias and chance, we should ask of a study that it be replicated and confirmed in other samples and other settings.

Summary

Confounding bias, chance, and causation – these are the three basic notions that underlie statistics and epidemiology. If clinicians understand these three concepts, then they will be able to believe their eyes more validly.

3 Levels of evidence

With a somewhat ready assumption of cause and effect and, equally, a neglect of the laws of chance, the literature becomes filled with conflicting cries and claims, assertions and counterassertions.

Austin Bradford Hill (Hill, 1962; p. 4)

The term *evidence* has become about as controversial as the word "unconscious" had been in the Freudian heyday, or as the term "proletariat" was in another arena. It means many things to many people, and for some, it elicits reverent awe – or reflexive aversion. This is because, like the other terms, it is linked to a movement – in this case evidence-based medicine (EBM) – which is currently quite influential and, with this influence, has attracted both supporters and critics.

This book is not about EBM per se, nor is it simply an application of EBM, although it is, in my view, consistent with EBM, rightly understood. I will expand on that topic further in Chapter 12, but for now, I would like to emphasize at the very start what I take to be the most important feature of EBM: the concept of *levels of evidence*.

Origins of EBM

It may be worthwhile to note that the originators of the EBM movement in Canada (such as David Sackett) toyed with different names for what they wanted to do; they initially thought about the phrase "science-based medicine" but opted for the term evidence instead. This is perhaps unfortunate since science tends to engender respect, while evidence seems a more vague concept. Hence we often see proponents of EBM (mistakenly, in my view) saying things like: "That opinion is not evidence-based" or "Those articles are not evidence-based." The folly of this kind of language is evident if we use the term "science" instead: "That opinion is not science-based" or "Those articles are not science-based." Once we use the term science, it becomes clear that such statements beg the question of what science means. Most of us would be open to such a discussion (which I touched on in the introduction). Yet (ironically perhaps due to the success of the EBM movement) many use the term "evidence" without pausing to think what it means. If some study is not "evidence-based," then what is it? "Non-evidence" based? "Opinion" based? But is there such a thing as "non-evidence"? Is there no opinion in evidence? Stated otherwise, do the facts speak for themselves? We have seen that they do not, which tells us that those who say such things as "That study is not evidence-based" are basically revealing their positivism: they could just as well say "That study is not science-based" because they have a very specific meaning in mind for science, which is in fact positivism. Since positivism is false, this extreme and confused notion of evidence is also false.

Table 3.1 Levels of evidence

Level I: Double-blind randomized trials
Ia: Placebo-controlled monotherapy
Ib: Non placebo-controlled comparison trials, or placebo-controlled add-on therapy trials
Level II: Open randomized trials
Level III: Observational studies
IIIa: Nonrandomized, controlled studies
IIIb: Large nonrandomized, uncontrolled studies (n > 100)
IIIc: Medium-sized nonrandomized, uncontrolled studies (100 > n > 50)
Level IV: Small observational studies (nonrandomized, uncontrolled, 50 > n > 10)
Level V: Case series (n < 10), *Case report* (n = 1), *Expert opinion*

From Soldani *et al.* (2005), with permission from Blackwell Publishing.

There is no inherent opposition between evidence and opinion, because "evidence" if meant to be "facts" always involves interpretation (which involves opinions or subjective assessments) as we discussed earlier.

In other words, all opinions are types of evidence; any perspective at all is based on some kind of evidence: there is no such thing as non-evidence.

In my reading of EBM, the basic idea is that we need to understand what kinds of evidence we use, and we need to use the best kinds we can: this is the concept of *levels* of evidence. Evidence-based medicine is *not* about an opposition between having evidence or not having evidence; it is about ranking different kinds of evidence (since we always have some kind of evidence or another).

Specific levels of evidence

The EBM literature has various definitions of specific levels of evidence. The main EBM text uses letters (A through D). I prefer numbers (1 through 5), and I think the specific content of the levels should vary depending on the field of study. The basic constant idea is that randomized studies are higher levels of evidence than non-randomized studies, and that the lowest level of evidence consists of case reports, expert opinion, or the consensus of the opinion of clinicians or investigators.

Levels of evidence provide clinicians and researchers with a road map that allows consistent and justified comparison of different studies so as to adequately compare and contrast their findings. Various disciplines have applied the concept of levels of evidence in slightly different ways, and in psychiatry, no consensus definition exists. In my view, in mental health, the following five levels of evidence best apply (Table 3.1), ranked from level I as highest and level V as lowest.

The key feature of levels of evidence to keep in mind is that each level has its own strengths and weaknesses, and, as a result, no single level is completely useful or useless. All other things being equal, however, as one moves from level V to level I, increasing rigor and probable scientific accuracy occurs.

Level V means a case report or a case series (a few case reports strung together), or an expert's opinion, or the consensus of experts or clinicians or investigators' opinions (such as in treatment algorithms), or the personal clinical experience of clinicians, or the words of wisdom of Great Professors (such as Freud or Kraepelin or Galen or Marx or Adam Smith). All of this is the same level of evidence: the lowest. This does not mean that such evidence is wrong, nor does it mean that it is *not* evidence; it *is* a kind of evidence, just a weak kind. It could turn out that a case report is correct, and a randomized study wrong, but, in general, randomized studies are much more likely to be correct than case reports. We simply cannot know when a case report, or an expert opinion, or a saying of Freud or Marx, is right, and when it is wrong. More often than not, such cases or opinions are wrong rather than right, but this does not mean that any single case or opinion might not, in fact, be correct. Authority is not, as with Rome, the last word.

All of medicine functioned on level V until the revolutionary work of Pierre Louis (1835), whose numerical method introduced level IV, the small observational study. How small is small? This will vary based on the topic of study, but one approach might be to say that a moderate effect size in clinical psychiatry requires two groups with samples of about 25 each for detection with p-values; hence a sample smaller than 50 might be considered "small"; for other disciplines and other outcomes, different numbers might be considered small: for instance, in clinical genetics, thousands of patients are required to detect the generally small genetic effect sizes being measured – thus 100 might be considered a small sample in that field. (See my discussion of the central limit theorem below.)

Observational studies are not randomized, and are open-label. Level III is the large observational study, such as the cohort study, the staple of the field of epidemiology. Here we would place such large and highly informative studies as the Framingham Heart Study, the Nurses Health Study, and so on. In those cases, the large samples involve more than a thousand patients. One might say in psychiatry that even greater than 50–100 might be considered large depending on the effect sizes being measured. Such observational studies (in this level as well as level IV) can be prospective or retrospective, with prospective studies being considered more valid (thus one might label them IIIa as opposed to IIIb for retrospective studies) due to the a-priori specification of outcomes as well as the usual careful rating and assessment of outcomes (as opposed to retrospective assessment of outcomes as is commonly the case in chart reviews, for instance).

Levels II and I take us to the highest levels of evidence due to randomization, which, as we saw, is the best tool to minimize or remove confounding bias (Chapter 2). Level II represents open (not double-blind) randomized clinical trials (RCTs) and level I represents double-blind RCTs. Within each level one might subgroup for small studies (in psychiatry < 50 subjects; IIb or Ic) versus large studies (> 50 subjects; IIa or Ib), and within level I studies, we might also subgroup based on use of placebo in large studies (Ia, the highest level of evidence).

Judging between conflicting evidence

The recognition of levels of evidence allows one to have a guiding principle by which to assess a literature. Basic rules are: 1. All other things being equal, a study at a higher level of evidence provides more valid (or powerful) results than one at a lower level. 2. Base judgments as much as possible on the highest levels of evidence. 3. Levels II and III are often the highest level of evidence attainable for complex conditions, and are to be valued in those circumstances. 4. Higher levels of evidence do not guarantee certainty; any one study can be wrong, thus look for replicability. 5. Within any level of evidence, studies may conflict based on other methodological issues not captured by the parameters used to provide the general outlines of levels of evidence.

One major advantage of a levels of evidence approach to an examination of data is that there is not a huge leap between double-blind, placebo-controlled studies and other, less rigorous levels. In other words, clinicians and some academics sometimes imagine that all studies that are not level I, double-blind RCTs, are equivalent in terms of rigor, accuracy, reliability, and information. In reality, there are many intermediate levels of evidence, each with particular strengths as well as limits. Open randomized studies and large observational studies, in particular, can be extremely informative and sometimes as accurate as level I studies. The concept of levels of evidence can also help clinicians who are loath to rely on level I controlled clinical trials, especially if those results contradict their own level V, clinical experiences. While the advantages to level V data mainly revolve around hypothesis generation, to devalue higher levels of evidence is unscientific and dangerous.

In my view, the concept of levels of evidence is the key concept of EBM. With it, EBM is valuable; without it, EBM is misunderstood.

Bias

4 Types of bias

> What the doctor saw with one, two, or three patients may be both acutely noted and
> accurately recorded; but what he saw is not necessarily related to what he did.
>   Austin Bradford Hill (Hill, 1962; p. 4)

The issue of bias is so important that it deserves even more clarification than the discussion
I gave in Chapter 2. In this chapter, I will examine the two basic types of bias: confounding
and measurement biases.

Confounding bias

To restate, the basic notion of confounding bias was shown in Figure 2.1, the "eternal triangle"
of the epidemiologist.

The idea is that we cannot believe our eyes; that in the course of observation, other factors of which we may not be aware (confounding factors) could be influencing our results.
The associations we think are happening (between treatment and outcome, or exposure and
result) may be due to something else altogether. We have constantly to be skeptical about
what we think we see; we have to be aware of, and even expect, that what seems to be happening is not really happening at all. The truth lies below the surface of what is observed: the
"facts" cannot be taken at face value.

Put in epidemiological language: "Confounding in its ultimate essence is a problem with
a particular estimate – a question of whether the magnitude of the estimate at hand could be
explained in terms of some *extraneous* factor" (Miettinen and Cook, 1981). And again: "By
'extraneous factor' is meant something other than the exposure or the illness – a characteristic
of the study subjects or of the process of securing information on them" (Miettinen and Cook,
1981).

Confounding bias is handled either by *preventing* it, through randomization in *study
design*, or by *removing* it, through regression models in *data analysis*. Neither option is guar-
anteed to remove all confounding bias from a study, but randomization is much closer to
being definitive than regression (or any other statistical analysis, see Chapter 5): one can better prevent confounding bias than remove it after the fact.

Another way of understanding the cardinal importance of confounding bias is to recognize that all medical research is about getting at the truth about some topic, and to do so one
has to make an unbiased assessment of the matter at hand. This is the basic idea that underlies
what A. Bradford Hill called "the philosophy of the clinical trial." Here is how this founder
of modern epidemiology explained the matter:

> …The reactions of human beings to most diseases are, under any circumstances,
> extremely variable. They do not all behave uniformly and decisively. They vary, and
> that is where the trouble begins. 'What the doctor saw' with one, two, or three patients

may be both acutely noted and accurately recorded; but *what he saw is not necessarily related to what he did*. The assumption that it is so related, with a handful of patients, perhaps mostly recovering, perhaps mostly dying, must, not infrequently, give credit where no credit is due, or condemn when condemnation is unjust. The field of medical observation, it is necessary to remember, is often narrow in the sense that no one doctor will treat many cases in a short space of time; it is wide in the sense that a great many doctors may each treat a few cases. Thus, with a somewhat ready assumption of cause and effect, and, equally, a neglect of the laws of chance, the literature becomes filled with conflicting cries and claims, assertions and counterassertions. It is thus, for want of an adequately controlled test, that various forms of treatment have, in the past, become unjustifiably, even sometimes harmfully, established in everyday medical practice … It is this belief, or perhaps state of unbelief, that has led in the last few years to a wider development in therapeutics of the more deliberately experimental approach.

(Hill, 1962; pp. 3–4; my italic)

Hill is referring to bloodletting and all that Galenic harm that doctors had practiced since Christ walked the earth. It is worth emphasizing that those who cared about statistics in medicine were interested as much, if not more, in disproving what doctors actually *do*, rather than proving what doctors *should* do. We cause a lot of harm, we always have, as clinicians, and we likely still are. The main reason for this morally compelling fact is this phenomenon of confounding bias. We know not what we do, yet we think we know.

This is the key implication of confounding bias, that we think we know things are such-and-such, but in fact they are not. This might be called *positive* confounding bias: the idea that there is a fact (drug X improves disease Y) when that fact is wrong. But there is also another kind of confounding bias; it may be that we think certain facts do not exist (say, a drug does not cause problem Z), when that fact does exist (the drug does cause problem Z). We may not be aware of the fact because of confounding factors which hide the true relationship between drug X and problem Z from our observation: this is called *negative* confounding bias.

We live in a confounded world: we never really know whether what we observe actually is happening as it seems, or whether what we fail to observe might actually be happening.

Let us see examples of how these cases play out in clinical practice

---

Clinical example 1 Confounding by indication: antidepressant discontinuation in bipolar depression

Confounding by indication (also called selection bias) is the type of confounding bias of which clinicians may be aware, though it is important to point out that confounding bias is not just limited to clinicians selecting patients non-randomly for treatment. There can also be other factors that influence outcomes of which clinicians are entirely unaware, or which clinicians do not influence at all (e.g, patients' dietary or exercise habits, gender, race, socioeconomic status). Confounding by indication, though, refers to the fact that, as mentioned in Chapter 2, *clinicians practice medicine non-randomly*: we do not haphazardly (one hopes) give treatments to patients; we seek to treat some patients with some drugs, and other patients with other drugs, based on judgments about various predictive factors (age, gender, type of illness, kinds of current symptoms, past side effects) that we think will maximize the chances that the patient will respond to the treatments we provide. The better we are in this process, the better our patients do, and the better clinicians we are. However, being a good clinician means that we will be bad researchers. If we conclude from our clinical successes that the treatments we use are quite effective, we may be mistaking the potency of our pills for our own clinical skills. Good outcomes simply mean that we know how to match patients to treatments; it does not mean that the treatments, in themselves or in general, are effective. To really know what the treatments do, we need to disentangle what we do, as clinicians, from what the pills do, as chemicals.

An example of likely confounding by indication from the psychiatric literature follows: An observational study of antidepressant discontinuation in bipolar disorder (Altshuler *et al.*, 2003) found that after initial response to a mood stabilizer plus an antidepressant, those who stayed on the combination stayed well longer than those in whom the antidepressant was stopped. In other words, at face value, the study seems to show that long-term continuation of antidepressants in bipolar disorder appears to lead to better outcomes. This study was published in the *American Journal of Psychiatry* (AJP) without any further statistical analysis, and this apparent result was discussed frequently at conferences for years subsequent to its publication.

But the study does not pass the first test of the Three C's. The first question, and one never asked by the peer reviewers of AJP (see Chapter 15 for a discussion of peer review), is whether there might be any confounding bias in this observational study.

Readers should begin to assess this issue by putting themselves in the place of the treating clinicians. Why would one stop the antidepressant after acute recovery? There is a literature that suggests that antidepressants can cause or worsen rapid-cycling in patients with bipolar disorder. So if a patient has rapid-cycling illness, some clinicians would be inclined to stop the antidepressant after acute recovery. If a patient had a history of antidepressant-induced mania that was common or severe, some clinicians might not continue the antidepressant. Perhaps if the patient had bipolar disorder type I, some clinicians would be less likely to continue antidepressants than if the patient had bipolar disorder type II. These are issues of selection bias, or so called confounding by indication: the doctor decides what to do non-randomly. Another way to frame the issue is this: we don't know how many patients did worse because they were taken off antidepressants versus how many were taken off because they were doing worse. There may also be other confounders that just happen to be the case: there may be more males in one group, a younger age of onset in one group, or a greater severity of illness in one group. To focus only on the potential confounding factor of rapid-cycling, if the group in whom antidepressant was stopped had more rapid cyclers (due to confounding by indication) than the other group (in whom the antidepressant was continued), then the observed finding that the antidepressant discontinuation group relapsed earlier than the other group would be due to the natural history of rapid-cycling illness: rapid cyclers relapse more rapidly than non-rapid cyclers. This would then be a classic case of confounding bias, and the results would have nothing to do with the antidepressants.

It may not be, in fact, that any of these potential confounders actually influenced the results of the study. However, the researchers and readers of the literature should think about and examine such possibilities. The authors of such studies usually do so in an initial table of demographic and clinical characterisitics (often referred to as "Table One" because it is needed in practically every clinical study, see Chapter 5). The first table should generally be a comparison of clinical and demographic variables in the groups being studied to see if there are any differences, which then might be confounders. For instance, if 50% of the antidepressant continuation group had rapid-cycling and so did 50% of the discontinuation group, then such confounding effects would be unlikely, because both groups are equally exposed. The whole point of randomized studies is that randomization more or less guarantees that all variables will be 50–50 distributed *across* groups (the key point is equal representation *across* groups, no matter what the absolute value of each variable is *within* each group, i.e., 5% vs. 50% vs. 95%). In an observational study, one needs to look at each variable one by one. If such possible confounders are identified, the authors then have two potential solutions: stratification or regression models (see below).

It is worth emphasizing that the baseline assessment of potential confounders in two groups has nothing to do with p-values. A common mistake is for researchers to compare two groups, note a p-value above 0.05, and then conclude that there is "no difference" and thus no confounding effect. However, such use of p-values is generally thought to be inappropriate, as will be discussed further below, because such comparisons are usually not the primary purpose of the study (the study might be focused on antidepressant outcome, not age or gender differences between groups). In addition, such studies are underpowered to detect many clinical and demographic differences (that is they have an unacceptably high possibility of a false negative or type II error), and thus p-value comparisons are irrelevant.

Perhaps the most important reason that p-values are irrelevant here is that any notable difference, even if not statistically significant, in a confounding factor (e.g., severity of illness), may have a major impact on an apparently statistically significant result with the experimental variable (e.g., antidepressant efficacy). Such a confounding effect may be big enough to completely swamp, or at least lessen the difference on the experimental variable such that a previously statistically significant (but small to moderate in effect size) result is no longer statistically significant. How large can such confounding effects be? The general rule of 10% or larger, *irrespective of statistical significance*, seems to hold (see Chapter 9). The major concern is not whether there is a statistically significant difference in a potential confounder, but rather whether there is a difference big enough to cause concern that our primary results may be distorted.

Clinical example 2   Positive confounding: antidepressants and post-stroke mortality

An example of standard confounding, another that went unnoticed in the AJP, is perhaps a bit tricky because it occurred in the setting of a randomized clinical trial (RCT). How can you have confounding bias in RCTs, the reader might ask? After all, RCTs are supposed to remove confounding bias. Indeed, this is so if RCTs are successful in randomization, i.e., if the two groups are equal on all variables being assessed in relation to the outcome being reported. However, there are at least two major ways that even RCTs can have confounding bias: first, they may be small in size and thus not succeed in producing equalization of groups by randomization (see Chapter 5); second, they may be unequal in groups on potential confounding factors in relation to the *outcome* being reported (i.e., on a secondary outcome, or a post-hoc analysis, even though the primary outcome might be relatively unbiased, see Chapter 8).

Here we have a study of 104 patients randomly given 12 weeks double-blind treatment of nortriptyline, fluoxetine, or placebo soon after stroke (Jorge *et al.*, 2003). According to the study abstract: "Mortality data were obtained for all 104 patients 9 years after initiation of the study." In those who completed the 12-week study, 48% had died in follow-up, but more of the antidepressant group remained alive (68%) than placebo (36%, p = 0.005). The abstract concludes: "Treatment with fluoxetine or nortriptyline for 12 weeks during the first 6 months post stroke significantly increased the survival of both depressed and nondepressed patients. This finding suggests that the pathophysiological processes determining the increased mortality risk associated with poststroke depression last longer than the depression itself and can be modified by antidepressants."

Now this is quite a claim: if you have a stroke and are depressed, only three months of treatment with antidepressants will keep you alive longer for up to a decade. The observation seems far-fetched biologically, but it did come from an RCT; it should be valid.

Once one moves from the abstract to the paper, one begins to see some questions rise up. As with all RCTs (Chapter 8), the first question is whether the results being reported were the primary outcome of the clinical trial; in other words, was the study designed to answer this question (and hence adequately powered and using p-values appropriately)? Was this study designed to show that if you took antidepressants for a few months after stroke, you would be more likely to be alive a decade later? Clearly not. The study was designed to show that antidepressants improved depression 3 months after stroke. This paper, published in AJP in 2003, does not even report the original findings of the study (not that it matters); the point is that one gets the impression that this study (of 9-year mortality outcomes) stands on its own, as if it had been planned all along, whereas the more clear way of reporting the study would have been to say that after a 3 month RCT, the researchers decided to check on their patients a decade later to examine mortality as a post-hoc outcome (an outcome they decided to examine long after the study was over). Next one sees that the researchers had reported only the completer results in the abstracts (i.e., those who had completed the whole 12-week initial RCT), which, as is usually the case, are more favorable to the drugs than the intent-to-treat (ITT) analysis (see Chapter 5 for discussion of why ITT is more valid). The ITT analysis still showed benefit but less robustly (59% with antidepressants vs. 36% with placebo, $p = 0.03$).

We can focus on this result as the main finding, and the question is whether it is valid. We need to ask the confounding question: were the two groups equal in all factors when followed up to 9-year outcome? The authors compared patients who died in follow-up (n = 50) versus those who lived (n = 54) and indeed they found differences (using a magnitude of difference of 10% between groups, see Chapter 5) in hypertension, obesity, diabetes, atrial fibrillation, and lung disease. The researchers only conducted statistical analyses correcting for diabetes, but not all the other medical differences, which could have produced the outcome (death) completely unrelated to antidepressant use. Thus many unanalyzed potential confounding factors exist here. The authors only examined diabetes due to a mistaken use of p-values to assess confounding and this mistake was pointed out in a letter to the editor (Sonis, 2004). In the authors' reply we see their lack of awareness of the major risk of confounding bias in such post-hoc analyses, even in RCTs: "This was not an epidemiological study; our patients were randomly assigned into antidepressant and placebo groups. The logic of inference differs greatly between a correlation (epidemiological) study and an experimental study such as ours." Unfortunately not. Assuming that randomization effectively removes most confounding bias (see Chapter 5), the logic of inference only differs between the primary outcome of a properly conducted and analyzed RCT and observational research (like epidemiological studies); but the logic of inference is the same for secondary outcomes and post-hoc analyses of RCTs as it is for observational studies. What is that logic? The logic of the need for constantly being aware of, and seeking to correct for, confounding bias.

One should be careful here not to be left with the impression that the key difference is between primary and secondary outcomes; the key issue is that with any outcome, but especially secondary ones, one should pay attention to whether confounding bias has been adequately addressed.

Clinical example 3 Negative confounding: substance abuse and antidepressant-associated mania

The possibility of negative confounding bias is often underappreciated. If one only looks at each variable in a study, one by one (univariate), compared to an outcome, each one of them might be unassociated; but, if one puts them all into a regression model, so that confounding effects between the variables are controlled, then some of them might turn out to be associated with the outcome (see Chapter 6).

Here is an example from our research on the topic of substance abuse as a predictor of antidepressant-related mania (ADM) in bipolar disorder. In the previous literature, one study had found such an association with a direct univariate comparison of substance abuse and the outcome of ADM (Goldberg and Whiteside, 2002). No regression modeling was conducted. We decided to try to replicate this study in a new sample of 98 patients, using regression models to adjust for confounding factors (Manwani *et al.*, 2006). In our initial analysis, with a simple univariate comparison of substance abuse and ADM, we found no link at all: ADM occurred in 20.7% of substance use disorder (SUD) subjects and 21.4% of non-SUD subjects. The relative risk (RR) was almost exactly the null value, with confidence intervals (CIs) symmetrical about the null (RR = 0.97, 95% CIs 0.64, 1.48). There was just no effect at all. If we had reported our result analyzed exactly as the previous study, the scientific literature would have existed of two identically designed conflicting results. This is quite common in observational studies, which are rife with confounding bias in all directions. Our study would have been publishable at that step, like so many others, and it would have just added one more confounded result to the psychiatric literature. However, after we conducted a multivariate regression, and thereby adjusted the effect of substance abuse for multiple other variables, not only did we observe a relationship between substance abuse and ADM, but it was an effect size of about threefold increased risk (odds ratio = 3.09, 95% CIs 0.92, 10.40). The wide CIs did not allow us to rule out the null hypothesis with 95% certainty, but they were definitely skewed in the direction of a highly probable positive effect.

Effect modification

An important concept to distinguish from confounding bias is effect modification (EM), which is related to confounding in that in both cases the relationship between the exposure (or treatment) and the outcome is affected. The difference is really conceptual. In confounding bias, the exposure really has no relation to the outcome at all; it is only through the confounding factor that any relation exists. Another way of putting this is that in confounding bias, the confounding factor causes the outcome; the exposure does not cause the outcome at all. The confounding factor is not on the causal pathway of an exposure and outcome. In other words, it is not the case that the exposure causes the outcome through the mediation of the confounding factor; the confounding factor is not merely a mechanism whereby the exposure causes the outcome. To repeat a classic example, numerous epidemiological studies find an association between coffee drinking and cancer, but this is due to the confounding effect of cigarette smoking: more coffee drinkers smoke cigarettes, and it is the cigarettes, completely and entirely, that cause the cancer; coffee itself has not increased cancer risk. This is confounding bias.

Let us suppose that the risk of cancer is higher in women smokers than in men smokers; this is no longer confounding bias, but EM. There is some interaction between gender and cigarette smoking, such that women are more prone biologically to the harmful effects of cigarettes (this is a hypothetical example). But we have no reason to believe that being female per se leads to cancer, as opposed to being male. Gender itself does not cause cancer; it is not a confounding factor; it merely modifies the risk of cancer with the exposure, cigarette smoking.

We might then contrast the differences between confounding bias and EM by comparing Figure 2.1 with Figure 4.1.

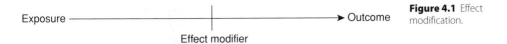

Figure 4.1 Effect modification.

When a variable affects the relationship between exposure and outcome, then a conceptual assessment needs to be made about whether the third variable directly causes the outcome but is not caused by the exposure (then it is a confounding factor), or whether the third variable does not cause the exposure and seems to modify the exposure's effects (then it is an effect modifier). In either case, those other variables are important to assess so that we can get a more valid understanding of the relationship between the exposures of interest and outcomes. Put another way, there is no way that a simple one-to-one comparison (as in univariate analyses) gives us a valid picture of what is really happening in observational experience. Both confounding bias and EM occur a lot, and they need to be assessed in statistical analyses.

Measurement bias

The other major type of bias, less important than confounding, is measurement bias. Here the issue is whether the investigator or the subject measures, or assesses, the outcome validly. The basic idea is that in subjective outcomes (such as pain), the subject or investigator might be biased in favor of what is being studied. In more objective outcomes (such as mortality), this bias will be less likely. Blinding (single – of the subject, double – of the subject and investigator) is used to minimize this bias.

Many clinicians mistake blinding for randomization. It is not uncommon for authors to write about "blinded studies" without informing us whether the study was randomized or not. In practice, blinding always happens with randomization (it is impossible to have a double-blind but then non-randomly decide about treatments to be given). However, it does not work the other way around. One can randomize, and not blind a study (open randomized studies) and this can be legitimate. Thus, blinding is optional; it can be present or not, depending on the study; but randomization is essential: it is what marks out the least biased kind of study.

If one has a "hard" outcome, such as death or stroke, where patients and subjects really cannot influence the outcomes based on their subjective opinions, blinding is not a key feature of RCTs. On the other hand, most psychiatric studies have "soft" outcomes, such as changes on symptom rating scales, and in such settings blinding is important.

Just as one needs to show that randomization is *successful* (see Chapter 5), one ought to show that blinding has been successful during a study. This would entail assessments by investigators and subjects of their best guess (usually at the end of a study) regarding which treatment (e.g., drug vs. placebo) was received. If the guesses are random, then one can conclude that blinding was successful; if the guesses correlate with the actual treatments given, then potential measurement bias can be present.

This matter is rarely studied. In one example, a double-blind study of alprazolam versus placebo for anxiety disorder, researchers assessed 129 patients and investigators about the allocated treatment after 8 weeks of treatment (Basoglu *et al.*, 1997). The investigators guessed alprazolam correctly in 82% of cases and they guessed placebo correctly in 78% of cases. Patients guessed correctly in 73% and 70% of cases respectively. The main predictor of correct guessing was presence of side effects. Treatment response did not predict correct guessing of blinded treatment.

If this study is correct, blinded studies really reflect about 20–30% blinding; otherwise patients and researchers make correct estimations and may bias results, at least to some extent. This unblinding effect may be strongest with drugs that have notable side effects.

A contemporary example might be found in recent randomized studies of quetiapine for acute bipolar depression (which led to a US Food and Drug Administration [FDA] indication). That drug was found effective in doses of 300 mg/d or higher, which produced sedation in about one-half of patients (Calabrese *et al.*, 2005). Given the much higher rate of sedation with this drug than placebo, the question can legitimately be asked whether this study was at best only partially blinded.

Measurement bias also comes into play in *not* noticing side effects. For instance, when serotonin reuptake inhibitors (SRIs) were first developed, early clinical trials did not have rating scales for sexual function. Since that side effect was not measured explicitly, it was underreported (people were reluctant to discuss sex). Observational experience identified much more sexual dysfunction than had been mistakenly reported in the early RCTs, and this clinical experience was confirmed by later RCTs that used specific sexual function rating scales.

Measurement bias is also sometimes called misclassification bias, especially in observational studies, when outcomes are inaccurately assessed. For instance, it may be that we conduct a chart review of whether antidepressants cause mania, but we had assessed manic symptoms unsystematically (e.g., rating scales for mania are not used usually in clinical practice), and then we recorded those assessments poorly (the charts might be messy, with brief notes rather than extensive descriptions). With such material, it is likely that at least mild hypomanic or manic episodes would be missed and reported as not existing. The extent of such misclassification bias can be hard to determine.

Chapter 5

Randomization

Experimental observations can be seen as experience carefully planned in advance.
Ronald Fisher (Fisher, 1971 [1935]; p. 8)

The most effective way to solve the problem of confounding is by the study design method of *randomization*. This is simply stated, but I would venture to say that this simple statement is the most revolutionary and profound discovery of modern medicine. I would include all the rest of medicine's discoveries in the past century – penicillin, heart transplants, kidney transplants, immunosuppression, gene therapies, all of it – and I would say that all of these specific discoveries are less important than the general idea, the revolutionary idea, of randomization, and this is so because without randomization, most of the rest of medicine's discoveries would not have been discovered: it is the power of randomization that allows us, usually, to differentiate the true from the false, a real breakthrough from a false claim.

Counting

I previously mentioned that medical statistics was founded on the groundbreaking study of Pierre Louis, in Paris of the 1840s, when he counted about 70 patients and showed that those with pneumonia who received bleeding died sooner than those who did not. Some basic facts – such as the fallacy of bleeding, or the benefits of penicillin – can be established easily enough by just counting some patients. But most medical effects are not as huge as the harm of bleeding or the efficacy of penicillin. We call those "large effect sizes": with just 70 patients one can easily show the benefit or the harm. Most medical effects, though, are smaller: they are medium or small effect sizes, and thus they can get lost in the "noise" of confounding bias. Other factors in the world can either obscure those real effects, or make them appear to be present when they are not.

How can we separate real effects from the noise of confounding bias? This is the question that randomization answers.

The first RCT: the Kuala Lumpur insane asylum study

A historical pause may be useful here. Ronald Fisher is usually credited with originating the concept of randomization. Fisher did so in the setting of agricultural studies in the 1920s: certain fields randomly received a certain kind of seed, others fields received other seeds. A. Bradford Hill is credited with adapting the concept to the first human randomized clinical trial (RCT), a study of streptomycin for pneumonia in 1948. Multiple RCTs in other conditions followed right away in the 1950s, the first in psychiatry involving lithium in 1952 and the antipsychotic chlorpromazine in 1954. This is the standard history, and it is correct in the sense that Fisher and Hill were clearly the first to formally develop the concept of randomization and to recognize its conceptual importance for statistics and science. But there is a hidden history, one that is directly relevant to the mental health professions.

As a historical matter, the first application of randomization in any scientific study appears to have been published by the American philosopher and physicist Charles Sanders Peirce in the late 1860s (Stigler, 1986). Peirce did not seem to follow up on his innovation however. Decades passed, and as statistical concepts began to seep into medical consciousness, it seems that the notion of randomization also began to come into being.

In 1905, in the main insane asylum of Kuala Lumpur, Malaysia, the physician William Fletcher decided to do an experiment to test his belief that white rice was *not*, as some claimed, the source of beriberi (Fletcher, 1907). He chose to do the study in the insane asylum because patients' diets and environment could be fully controlled there. He obtained the permission of the government (though not the patients), and lined up all of them, assigning consecutive patients to receive either white or brown rice. For one year, the two groups received identical diets except for the different types of rice. Fletcher had conducted the first RCT, and it occurred in psychiatric patients, in an assessment of diet (not drug treatment). Further, the result of the RCT refuted, rather than confirmed, the investigator's hypothesis: Fletcher found that beriberi happened in 24/120 (20%) who received white rice, versus only 2/123 (1.6%) who received brown rice. In the white rice diet group 18/120 (15%) died of beriberi, versus none in the brown rice diet group (Silverman, 1998). Fisher had not invented p-values yet, but if Fletcher had had access to them, he would have seen the chance likelihood of his findings was less than 1 in 1000 ($p < 0.0001$); as it was, he knew that the difference between 20% and 2% was large enough to matter.

Arguably, Fletcher had stumbled on the most powerful method of modern medical research. Since not all who ate white rice developed beriberi, the absolute effect size was not large enough to make it an obvious connection. But the relative risk (RR) was indeed quite large (applying modern methods, the RR was 12.3, which is slightly larger than the association of cigarette smoking and lung cancer; the 95% confidence intervals are 3.0 to 50.9, indicating almost total certitude of a threefold or larger effect size). It took randomization to clear out the noise and let the real effect be seen. At the same time, Fletcher had also discovered the method's premier capacity: its ability to disabuse us of our mistaken clinical observations.

Randomizing liberals and conservatives, blondes and brunettes

How do we engage in randomization?

We do it by randomly assigning patients to a treatment versus a control (such as placebo, or another treatment). You get drug, you get placebo, you get drug, you get placebo, and so on. By doing so randomly, after a large enough number of persons, we ensure that the two groups – drug and placebo – are equal in *all* factors except the experimental choice of receiving drug or placebo. There will be equal numbers of males and females in both groups, equal numbers of old and young persons, equal numbers of those with more severe illness and less severe illness – all the *known* potential confounding factors will be equal in both groups, and thus there will be no *differential* biasing effect of those factors on the results. But more: suppose it turns out in a century that hair color affects our results, or political affiliation, or something apparently ridiculous like how one puts on one's pants in the morning; still, there will be equal numbers of blondes and brunettes in both groups, and equal numbers of liberals and conservatives (we won't prejudge which group would have a worse outcome), and equal numbers of those who put their pants on left leg first versus right leg first in both groups. In other words, all the *unknown* potential confounding factors would also be equalized between both groups.

This is the power of randomization: *all* potential confounding factors – *known or unknown* – should be equalized between the groups, such that the results should be valid, *at face value, now and forever.* (One is tempted to add "Amen," which would be the chorus for proponents of ivory-tower evidence-based medicine [EBM], see Chapter 12.)

This is obviously the ideal situation; RCTs can be invalid, or less valid, due to multiple other design factors outside of randomization (see Chapter 8). But, if all other aspects of an RCT are well-designed, the impact of randomization is that it can provide something as close to absolute truth as is possible in the world of medical science.

Measuring success of randomization

All these claims are contingent on the RCT being well-designed. And the first matter of importance is that the randomization needs to be "successful," by which we mean that as best as we can tell, the two groups are in fact equal on almost all variables that we can measure. Usually this is assessed in a table (usually the first table in a paper, and thus often referred to as "Table One") comparing clinical and demographic characteristics of the two (or more) randomized subgroups in the overall sample.

The most important feature that differentiates whether randomization will be successful is *sample size*. This is by far the most important factor and it is easy to understand. Even before randomization as a concept was developed, the relevance of sample size for confounding bias was identified by a nineteenth-century founder of statistics, Quetelet, who wrote in 1835: "The greater the number of individuals observed, the more do individual peculiarities, whether physical or moral, become effaced, and allow the general facts to predominate, by which society exists and is preserved." (Stigler, 1986; p. 172.)

If I flip a coin twice, it might turn out heads–heads, or tails–tails rather frequently; I have to flip it lots of times for it to be close to 50% heads and 50% tails, as it will by chance. But how many times is "lots of times"? That is the question of sample size: how large does a study have to be to equalize confounding factors between groups reasonably well? Large enough to answer the question being asked, but this does not mean that all studies should be huge, or that larger is always better. At the very least, that attitude will have ethical problems, since many people may be unnecessarily exposed to research risks when a small number would have answered the question. With this background, as the saying goes: "A study needs to be as large as it needs to be." Not larger, and not smaller.

Put another way, we don't want a study to have unequal confounding factors in two groups despite randomizing patients to those two groups. This can happen by chance; just because we randomize, it does not follow that two groups will be equal in confounding factors. The more patients we randomize, however, the more likely that the two groups will be equal in confounding factors. The question is: how much more?

The central limit theorem

There are two ways to answer this question: one clinical and one mathematical.

Clinically, to limit ourselves to psychiatric research, given moderate effect sizes for often subjective variables (such as improvement in depressive symptom scores), one might generalize to say that at least 25 patients are needed per arm to detect a moderate effect size difference between groups. (Confounding factors could still impact the results, though.)

Mathematically, one might turn to the concept of the "central limit theorem." Stated mathematically, this means that "if you have an average, it should have a normal sampling distribution." In other words, the idea here is that if you obtain the average of a number of observations, then that average will be normally distributed after a certain number of observations. Getting back to our coin flip, two observations (flipping the coin just twice) is unlikely to give us a common average of 50% heads and 50% tails: the sample will not be normally distributed. On the other hand, 1000 observations will be normally distributed, with the most common observation being 50% likely heads and 50% likely tails, and infrequent observations of extremes in either direction (mostly heads or mostly tails). So the central limit theorem comes down to this: how many times do you have to flip a coin to get a normal distribution of observations (where the most common observation is 50% head and tails, and there are equal frequencies of observing either extreme)? The answer seems to be about n = 50.

Thus, whether clinically or mathematically, we come up with a figure of about 50 patients as being the cutoff for a large versus a small randomized study (hence the rationale for this figure in Table 3.1).

Interpreting small RCTs

If the sample size is too small (< 50), what are we to make of the RCT? In other words, if someone conducts a double-blind placebo-controlled RCT of 10 or 20 or 30 patients, what are we to make of it?

Basically, since it is highly likely that confounding factors will be unequal between groups, my view is that small RCTs should be seen as observational studies: they are perhaps slightly better in that they should not be *as* biased as a standard observational study, yet they *are* still biased. Hence, they cannot be taken at face value.

Even if a Table One showed that some measured variables are equal between groups in a small RCT, unmeasured confounders are still likely that could influence the results.

Also, because they are small, such RCTs cannot even be adequately assessed through statistical analyses, such as regression models, to reduce confounding bias (see Chapter 6). Their results simply have to stand on their own, as neither valid nor invalid, and as potentially meaningful, but equally potentially meaningless.

Two clinical examples of small RCTs

Here is an example of a small RCT that is possibly useful, but equally possibly meaningless. Researchers wanted to show that serotonin reuptake inhibitor (SRI) antidepressants were effective in type II bipolar disorder (Parker *et al.*, 2006). They gave citalopram by itself (without mood stabilizers) versus placebo to nine patients for 3 months; then those who had received one arm of treatment were switched to the other treatment for 3 months; then they were switched back again to the original treatment for another 3 months. The switching of treatments reflects a crossover design, but most relevant for our discussion is that the "randomization" initially involved four patients getting one treatment and five patients getting another. This obviously is nowhere near the number of repetitions that is required to equalize the two groups on most possible confounding factors. In the case of crossover studies, patients can, in a sense, serve as their own controls, as they are switched successively to drug versus placebo. So this study might have had more rationale than if it had been a simple parallel design study (e.g., four patients get drug versus five patients who get placebo, without any further changes). But even with the crossover component, a study of this size is somewhat of a *glorified observational study*, and thus benefit with the drug would only be somewhat more impressive than in an observational report.

Another example is a study I conducted with my colleagues, assessing efficacy of divalproex, an anticonvulsant, in acute bipolar depression (Ghaemi *et al.*, 2007). The clinical lore is that this drug is ineffective in this setting. Nineteen patients were used in total (half drug and half placebo) in a double-blind RCT, and we showed benefit. The study was not underpowered, that is, the small sample size did not lead to low statistical power, because our result was positive. Lack of statistical power is only relevant for negative studies (see Chapter 8). However, the positive result may have been biased by the small sample due to unsuccessful randomization, which is likely the case. Was the study worth doing?

The key is to avoid ivory-tower EBM (Chapter 12). One should not compare a study to the ideal design (all studies should then have one million patients and be triple-blind and placebo-controlled); one should compare a study to the best available evidence in the literature, asking the question: does the study advance our current knowledge? In this case, since there were only two prior small RCTs (one unpublished and negative, and one published and positive), our results at least push the literature a few inches in the positive direction.

One cannot infer definitive causation (see Chapter 10), but our study adds, albeit in a limited way, to our knowledge and would lead us to continue to seek to see if this drug works in this condition with more studies (while a negative study might have led to less rationale for further research on this topic).

"Table One"

I mentioned that success of randomization needs to be assessed by a "Table One" which compares clinical and demographic variables in the two randomized groups. Some key concepts are needed to construct and interpret such a table. First, such tables should *never* have p-values. This is because, as described in Chapter 8, RCTs are *not* designed to assess the relative frequency of males or females (or Republicans vs. Democrats, or a host of other potential confounding factors) in the two groups, RCTs are designed to answer some question like whether a drug is more effective than placebo. That is the hypothesis the study is designed to test, not the frequency of 100 potential confounding variables. If p-values are used, their being positive is meaningless (due to false positive results given multiple comparisons; see Chapter 7), and their being negative is meaningless (due to false negative results since the sample may be too small to detect small differences between groups; see Chapter 7). Thus, no p-values should be used at all in Table One to distinguish potential confounding factors between two groups. Without p-values, how are we then supposed to tell if the two groups differ enough in a variable such that it might exert a confounding effect? If a study has 51% males and 49% females, is that enough of a difference to be a confounding effect? What if it is 52% males, 48% females? 53% vs. 47%? 55% vs. 45%? Where is the cutoff where we should be concerned that randomization might have failed, that chance variation between groups on a variable might have occurred despite randomization?

The ten percent solution

Here is another part of statistics that is arbitrary: we say that a 10% difference between groups is the cutoff for a potential confounding effect. Thus, since 10% of 50 is 5%, we would be concerned about a gender difference that is something like 55% vs. 45% (plus or minus 5% from the median). Suppose 25% of one group in our sample had a history of hospitalization for the illness being studied (and thus could be seen as more severely ill than those without past hospitalization); if the other group had a 31% rate of past hospitalization, the difference between the two groups is 6%, and we would be concerned about a difference between the groups of even 3% (10% of the absolute rate, which is 25% in one group and 31% in another group, or around 30% overall), and thus we definitely would be concerned about the observed 6% difference between the groups in past hospitalization (31% – 25% = 6%). It may turn out, if we mistakenly did a p-value, that the p-value would be 0.22 (not statistically significant), but we do not care. This study was not designed or powered to differentiate the two groups on past hospitalization; this hypothesis was not made before the study was conducted; and thus a p-value hypothesis test for this difference is wrong to do. We just care about the absolute difference between the groups in this variable, and it is bigger than a 10% relative difference between the groups, and thus it is a potential confounding factor.

Then what do we do? We have a potential confounding factor; our study is over; we have the randomized results. How does this imbalance in our Table One influence our results?

There are at least two ways one can handle identified potential confounding bias after an RCT is finished. The most common approach is simply to report the randomized results as observed, state that there might be residual confounding bias as identified in Table One in relation to variable Y (gender, or past hospitalization), and thus to imply that the results need to be taken with a grain of salt: they have some risk of invalidity. The other approach would be to conduct a regression model with the variable in question included so as to see if the observed randomized results change or not (see Chapter 6). In other words, one could treat the RCT as if it was an observational study, and analyze it accordingly (with regression models). If there is no or minimal change in the randomized result, one could then say that the observed imbalance was minor and had no appreciable confounding effect on the randomized study outcomes.

Not all RCTs are created equal

The point of all this discussion is that, too often, researchers conduct a randomized study, and report the results, and that is it. They *assume* that randomization was successful (even though the study might be small, or even though there might in fact be observed imbalances in Table One). One should not assume the success of randomization, one should show it. *Not all RCTs are created equal.* Readers should be aware of this fact, and even though RCTs should be viewed as more likely valid than other studies, they are not automatically valid, and the success of randomization should always be the first question that is asked and answered before one begins to consider an RCT as potentially valid.

Chapter 6

Regression

Numbers do not lie, but they have the propensity to tell the truth with intent to deceive.

Eric Temple Bell (Salsburg, 2001; p. 234)

The best way to reduce confounding bias in observational studies is stratification or regression.

Stratification

Stratification means that one sees how patients do with and without the potential confounder. With the example of a study of whether a toxin causes cancer, it is important to know how many smokers and non-smokers there are in the sample. If the toxin causes the same cancer rate in smokers as it does in non-smokers, then you can conclude that smoking does not explain the results. Similarly, in a study of antidepressant treatment of bipolar disorder, for instance, one could assess the results in those with rapid-cycling and separately in those without rapid-cycling. If the survival curves all had the same results, then one could conclude that it would be unlikely that rapid-cycling was a confounder. The advantage of stratification is that it is easy to interpret and does not require complex statistics. The disadvantage is that one can really only look at one confounder at a time.

Stratification is a markedly underused method of addressing confounding bias (Rothman and Greenland, 1998). At a simple level, if two strata on a potential confounding factor (e.g., smoking) are the same, then that factor *cannot* confound one's results. Further, if a study does not contain any, or hardly any, persons with a potential confounding factor, then it *cannot* be confounded by that factor (this is called "restriction" as opposed to stratification).

One of the benefits of stratification, compared to regression, is that one does not need to make certain assumptions about whether the regression model can be applied to the data (see Appendix). The key weakness is that one cannot correct for multiple confounders simultaneously, but at least one can capture major confounders with this simple method. Also one can use stratification to do sensitivity analyses, looking at whether individual factors change one's results.

Regression

What if, as is usually the case, one thinks there might be multiple confounders? For instance, besides rapid-cycling, what if we are concerned about differences in severity of illness, or gender, age, or even things like the therapeutic alliance or patient compliance or other factors. Stratification does not handle more than one or a few confounders at a time. For multiple confounders, one has to use a mathematical model, called a *regression* model.

To ease the potential strangeness of such statistical language to clinicians, it is important to note that regression models basically represent the same thing (quantified) that clinicians do intuitively. When clinicians see patients, they conceive of patients in the whole complexity of the presentation. Thus, one patient might be an elderly obese male with medical illness and many side effects who has been ill for decades. Another patient might be a young thin female with no previous treatment and only a short period of illness. Even in these simple clinical descriptions, multiple factors (age, gender, duration of illness, past treatment response, weight) are intuitively taken into account by experienced clinicians as they make judgments about diagnosis and treatment. Regression models simply identify and quantify the effects of these clinical factors on outcome.

The key to regression is that it allows one to measure the experimental effect adjusted for some of the confounders. It also allows one to get the magnitude of effect of the various predictors on their own. The main disadvantage to regression models is that they do not control or adjust for confounders on which one may not have accurate or adequate data, nor do they adjust for potential confounders that are unknown at the time of the study. These latter problems are only addressed by randomization. But, in the setting of observational studies, regression modeling can reduce, though never completely remove, confounding bias.

Conflicting studies

A major reason why conflicting studies are present in the medical literature is that many of those studies are observational studies, and the vast majority make no effort to identify or correct for confounding bias. As Hill wrote, "One difficulty, in view of the variability of patients and their illnesses, is in classifying the patients into, at least, broad groups so that we may be sure that like is put with like, both before and after treatment." (Hill, 1971; p. 9.) When confounding bias is not assessed in observational studies, often like is not being compared with like, and all kinds of varying results will be reported.

Assessing confounding factors

How should one compare two groups to tell whether differences between them might reflect confounding bias? Two basic options exist: to use p-values, or simply to compare the magnitude of difference between the groups. Computer simulation models have compared these alternatives, and, all in all, the magnitude of difference approach seems most sensitive to detecting confounding effects. P-values are too coarse of a measure: they only capture major differences between groups (if they are used, the computer simulations suggest that they should be set at a high level, e.g., $p < 0.20$ would indicate a difference that could lead to potential confounding effects). However, two subgroups in a sample may have a moderate or even small difference on some factor, but if that factor has a major effect on the outcome, a confounding effect can happen. In the computer simulations, it was found that a low potential absolute difference between groups (such as 10%) predicted confounding effects rather well (see Chapter 5).

The meaning of "adjusted" data

In sum, the basic concept behind regression modeling is that we will control for all potential confounding variables. In other words, we will look at the results for the variable which interests us (one might call it the *experimental* variable), *while keeping all other variables fixed.* So, if we want to know if antidepressants cause mania, the outcome is mania, and the experimental variable is antidepressant use. If we want to remove the effect of other confounding variables – such as age, gender, age of onset, years ill, severity of depression, etc. – we will put those variables into a regression model. The mathematical equation of the regression model can be seen, in a way, as keeping all those other values fixed, so as to give a more accurate result for the experimental variable (antidepressant use). The outcome of looking at antidepressant use and mania without assessing other confounding variables is called the *unadjusted* or *crude* result. The outcome of assessing antidepressant use and mania while also controlling for other confounding variables is called the *adjusted* result. Another way of putting this process is that we are adjusting the results which appear to be the case at face value (the *crude* results) to make them closer to what they *really* are (or what they really would be seen to be in a randomized study, where the effect of all confounding variables is removed). If the crude (or unadjusted) and the adjusted results are not much different, then the variables included in the model did not have much confounding effects. In that case, the crude results can be seen as valid, unless, of course, one has failed to identify some variables which might be exerted confounding effects and are not adjusted in the regression model.

A conceptual defense of regression

Some people do not like the concept of adjustment, perhaps because it smacks of fiddling with the data: after all, the "real" results, what are actually observed, are being mathematically manipulated. Such critics fail to realize that *what one observes in the real world is often not what is really there*. This is another philosophical concept, which is simple to show to be true, at the basis of statistics. The sun appears to be about the size of my hand, but it is much larger. I have never seen an atom, but this apparently solid table is made of them. What appears to be the case is not all there is to reality. So it is with clinical observations in medicine. We think coffee causes cancer if we simply associate the two, but the coffee drinkers are smokers and the cause is the latter. If we do not assess smoking, and take it into account, the "real" observation of coffee and cancer will fool us.

Hence adjustment in regression models is perfectly legitimate, but the phrase can be altered if one likes to others, such as "controlling" for confounding factors, or "correcting" for confounding factors. Any of these terms are interchangeable: "adjusted" results, or results "controlled" or "corrected" for other variables.

Regression equations

The mathematical concept behind regression modeling is complex, but the basics are worth understanding, since often results are reported with the basic equation's terms.

If I want to know the probability of an association between an experimental predictor (as defined above) and an outcome, I can express it simply this way:

$$P\,(\text{Outcome}) = \beta\,(\text{Predictor})$$

$$\text{where P\,(Outcome)} = \text{the probability of the outcome}$$

$$\text{and } \beta\,(\text{Predictor}) = \text{the effect of the predictor.}$$

Beta is the variable for the effect size of the predictor, or how much the predictor impacts on the outcome.

As described in Chapter 9, effect sizes come in two varieties, absolute and relative. Absolute effect sizes are amounts, such as the difference between drug and placebo on a mood rating scale. If drug leads to 5 points more improvement on the rating scale than placebo, then the *absolute effect size* between the two treatments is 5. Effect size can also be relative. If 80% of those on drug improved markedly versus 20% of those on placebo, then the relative effect size is $80/20 = 4$. This is often called the *risk ratio*, a type of relative risk. Another kind of relative risk is the *odds ratio*, which is another way of expressing the risk ratio. While the straight risk ratio is a probability, the odds ratio is a measure of a fair bet that something will happen. Odds ratios and risk ratios are different, and as probabilities increase for risk ratios, odds ratios increase exponentially (see Chapter 9).

The relevance of this discussion is that the relative effect sizes that are obtained in regression models are odds ratios, not risk ratios, and thus we need to remember that huge odds do not represent absolute probabilities of that size. The equation for regression models involves logarithms, and the conversion of logarithms to effect sizes produces odds ratios, not risk ratios.

Multivariate regression

Back to our equation. We have a predictor and an outcome; this is an association which is direct and uncorrected for any potential confounding variables. In the phrasing of studies, this is a *univariate* analysis; only one predictor is assessed. We might be interested in two predictors, or we might want to adjust our results for one other variable besides our experimental variable. Our equation would then become:

$$P\,(\text{Outcome}) = \beta_1\,(\text{Predictor}_1) + \beta_2\,(\text{Predictor}_2)$$

where Predictor_1 is the experimental variable, and Predictor_2 is the second variable, which might be a confounding factor, or which might itself be a second predictor of the outcome. This equation is a *bivariate* analysis.

Sometimes researchers report bivariate analyses, comparing the experimental with the outcome, correcting for a single variable, *one after the other, separately*. This would be something like:

$$P\,(\text{Outcome}) = \beta_1\,(\text{Predictor}_1) + \beta_2\,(\text{Predictor}_2)$$
$$P\,(\text{Outcome}) = \beta_1\,(\text{Predictor}_1) + \beta_3\,(\text{Predictor}_3)$$
$$P\,(\text{Outcome}) = \beta_1\,(\text{Predictor}_1) + \beta_4\,(\text{Predictor}_4)$$
$$P\,(\text{Outcome}) = \beta_1\,(\text{Predictor}_1) + \beta_5\,(\text{Predictor}_5).$$

The problem with these bivariate analyses is that they will correct the experimental predictor for each one separately, but they do not correct it for *all variables together*. Let us suppose that the experimental predictor is coffee drinking and the outcome is cancer; and let us suppose that the main confounding factor is smoking but that this effect is primarily seen in older smokers rather than younger smokers. Thus, the confounding effect involves two variables: smoking and age. If Predictor_2 is smoking, and Predictor_3 is age, then this combined effect will be underestimated in serial bivariate equations. This effect can only be seen in multivariate analysis, where all the factors are included in one model:

$$P\,(\text{Outcome}) = \beta_1\,(\text{Predictor}_1) + \beta_2\,(\text{Predictor}_2) + \beta_3\,(\text{Predictor}_3)$$
$$+ \beta_4\,(\text{Predictor}_4) + \beta_5\,(\text{Predictor}_5).$$

The other benefit of multivariate analysis is that it not only corrects the effect size of the experimental variable $\beta_1\,(\text{Predictor}_1)$ for the other predictor variables, but it also *corrects all the predictor variables for each other*. Thus, if the estimate of the effect size of the impact

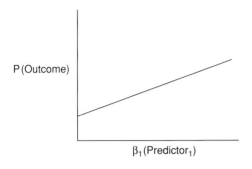

Figure 6.1 Outcome versus Predictor$_1$.

of smoking on cancer is confounded by age (higher in older persons and lower in younger persons), then the multivariate analysis will correct for age in the effect size that is estimated for the smoking variable.

Visualizing regression

We can now perhaps best proceed with understanding regression modeling by visualizing what it entails. Suppose the probability of the outcome – P (Outcome) – is on the y-axis, and on the x-axis we have the adjusted effect size (β value) of the experimental predictor.

The graph of this process would look something like Figure 6.1.

The slope of this line is the effect size, or β value, with the probability of the outcome varying.

Take the example of someone who is age 35 and has been ill with depression for 20 years, in whom we want to assess the efficacy of antidepressants (Predictor$_1$ is antidepressant use and the Outcome is being classified as a treatment responder); the equation would be:

$$P\,(\text{Outcome}) = \beta_1\,(\text{antidepressant use}) + \beta_2\,(\text{age}) + \beta_3\,(\text{years ill})$$

which would be

$$P\,(\text{Outcome}) = \beta_1\,(\text{antidepressant use}) + \beta_2\,(35) + \beta_3\,(20).$$

Another patient might have received antidepressant but with an age of 55 and 30 years ill, producing the equation:

$$P\,(\text{Outcome}) = \beta_1\,(\text{antidepressant use}) + \beta_2\,(55) + \beta_3\,(30).$$

In these cases, the calculation of the effect of antidepressant use, β_1, would be adjusted for, or corrected for, the changes in age and years ill between patients. In other words, β_1 would not change in the above two equations. It is as if the values for the effect of age (β_2) and years ill (β_3) were calculated at an average amount for all patients, or kept constant in all patients, thus removing any differences they might cause in the overall equation.

The differing patients above might be visualized as in Figure 6.2.

What is visually clear is that the slopes are always the same, that is, the effect size for the experimental predictor – β_1 (Predictor$_1$) – never changes. The change in the absolute result of the equation is only reflected in changes in the y-intercept, which is captured mathematically as β_0, a term which has no relevant clinical meaning, but which reflects the start of the curve that is being modeled with regression.

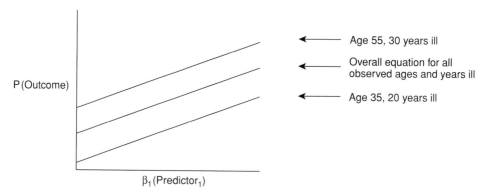

Figure 6.2 Outcome versus Predictor₁ adjusted for other predictors (e.g., age, years ill).

The equation of a multivariate regression model then ends up as follows:

$$P\,(\text{Outcome}) = \beta_0 + \beta_1\,(\text{Predictor}_1) + \beta_2\,(\text{Predictor}_2) + \beta_3\,(\text{Predictor}_3)$$
$$+ \beta_4\,(\text{Predictor}_4) + \beta_5\,(\text{Predictor}_5)\ldots$$

Not too many variables

The number of predictors can obviously not be infinite. Researchers need to define how many predictors or confounders need to be included in a regression model. How this process of choice occurs can be somewhat subjective, or it might be put into the hands of a computer model. In either case, some kind of decision must be made, often due to sample size limitations. Mathematically, the more variables are included in a regression model, the lower the statistical power of the analysis. This is referred to as *collinearity*, since frequently variables will correlate with each other (such as age and number of years ill), and thus multiple variables may in fact be assessing the same clinical predictor. Besides this factor, as noted above, multiple statistical comparisons always increase the risks of chance outcomes. (As noted below, this factor is perhaps the major limitation in regression modeling.) In other words, even if an experimental variable strongly impacts an outcome in a study of 100 patients, this strong result might be statistically significant in a univariate analysis, a bivariate analysis, or even a multivariate analysis with 5 variables. But if 15 variables are included, eventually, that p-value will rise above 0.05, and suddenly – poof, there is no result! We want to avoid saying there is no effect when there might indeed be one, and thus one should not include too many variables in a regression model. But how many is too many? Deciding which variables to include and which to exclude is a complex process. In the Appendix, I have provided detailed examples of how regression modeling can be conducted. Here I will only point out that the specifics of how regression can be conducted can often seem like a black box, and indeed they can be. One must rely on objectivity and care on the part of researchers. Some computerized methods can also help standardize the process (see Appendix).

Effect modification again

Readers should be reminded that interactions between predictors and other variables do not always reflect confounding effects; sometimes they reflect effect modification. As discussed in Chapter 4, this is where it is useful, even necessary, to be a clinician: to appreciate confounding bias versus effect modification, one needs to understand the condition and variables being studied. In confounding bias, the confounding variable *is* itself the causal source of the outcome; in effect modification, the effect modifier *is not* the causal source of the outcome (the experimental variable causes the outcome, but only through interaction with the effect modifier). The numbers alone cannot tell this story; the researcher needs to think about the illness.

Recall classic examples from medical epidemiology, repeated here from Chapter 4 so that this distinction is clear. Here is an example of effect modification: cigarette smoking frequently causes blood clots in women on birth control pills. Being female itself is not a cause of blood clots; nor do oral contraceptives themselves have a large risk; but those two variables (gender and oral contraceptive status) together increase this risk of cigarette smoking greatly. Contrast this example with confounding bias: coffee causes cancer; numerous epidemiological studies show this. Of course, it does not, because coffee drinking is higher among those who smoke cigarettes, and cigarette smoking (the confounding variable) is the cause of the cancer.

As discussed in the Appendix, then, interactions between experimental and other variables can be interpreted as confounding bias or effect modification mainly based on the knowledge of researchers, not primarily based on any quantitative measures.

Regression in RCTs

Up to now, to keep it simple, I have emphasized the use of regression modeling only for observational studies. In contrast, I have said that in clinical trials, they are not needed: since confounding bias is removed by the research design (randomization), there is no need to try to remove it by data analysis (regression modeling).

Some take this distinction too literally, thereby creating a fetish out of RCTs (randomized clinical trials). In fact, regression modeling should still be used even after RCTs are conducted as a mechanism of sensitivity analysis. In other words, did those RCTs in fact succeed in removing confounding bias? If they did, then regression models should not change any of the findings about the relationship between experimental variables and outcomes (unlike observational studies). If, however, regression models change some results, then either confounding bias or effect modification might be at work, and the RCT would need to be more carefully analyzed.

This is relevant because even though RCTs are *meant* to remove confounding bias by means of randomization, one cannot assume that they *succeed* in doing so. One cannot *assume* the success of randomization; one must *prove* it.

Chance

7 Hypothesis-testing: the dreaded p-value and statistical significance

> The p-value is a mathematical replacement for sensible thought.
>
> Alvan Feinstein (Feinstein, 1977)

Should we just stop using p-values?

Some might think that a statistics book that makes this claim would have nothing more to say. But in fact, it should be clear by now that there is much more to statistics than p-values (or hypothesis-testing methods). In fact, statistics has little to do with p-values, or, more correctly, p-values have as much to do with statistics as alcohol has to do with sociability: too much of the former ruins the latter.

Background

The concept of the p-value comes from Ronald Fisher, in his work on randomization of crops for agriculture. P-values are, in effect, a statistical attempt to solve the philosophical problem called *the problem of induction* (see Chapter 10). If we observe something, we can never be 100% absolutely certain that what we have observed actually happened. It is possible that other things influenced what we observed (confounding bias; this is perhaps the most important source of error in induction), and it is possible that we observed something that occurred by chance. As discussed more in Chapter 10, the philosopher David Hume had long identified this probabilistic nature of induction. We have seen that each day the sun rises, he said. Day after day, the sun rises. Yet we never have complete (absolute, 100%) certainty that the sun will rise tomorrow. It is highly, highly likely (one might say 99.99% probable) that the sun will rise tomorrow, and thus we can proceed with the inductive inference that the sun will rise tomorrow. However, this strong inference does not imply that we are absolutely certain that this will happen.

For practical purposes, the difference between 99.99% and 100% is unimportant. (For philosophical purposes it may matter, and much has been made about Hume's argument that one cannot infer absolute causation from induction.) Probably 99.98% is also close enough to 100% that it should not matter that there is a 0.02% risk that the event observed might have occurred by chance. What about 99.97%? 99.96%? 99.0%? 98%, 97%, 96%, 95%? Aha! We have reached the magic number. Or at least this is the number that is generally viewed as magic in contemporary research: the p-value of 0.05, which reflects a 95% likelihood that an observed inductive inference did not occur by chance.

Perhaps the reader can appreciate that the cutoff point of 95% vs. 96% or 94% or 99% is rather arbitrary. Fisher never states anywhere why he thinks the p-value of 0.05 is preferable to 0.06 or 0.04 or 0.01. Presumably, the number 5 is more pleasing to the eye than 4 or 6.

David Salsburg, a statistician who searched Fisher's articles and books for an origin to this concept, reports that he only finds one place (interestingly for mental health professionals, it occurred in the 1929 *Proceedings of the Society for Psychical Research*) where Fisher ascribes to the p = 0.05 criterion, and there Fisher is clear that the decision is arbitrary:

> In the investigation of living beings by biological methods, statistical tests of significance are essential. Their function is to prevent us being deceived by accidental occurrences, due not to the causes we wish to study, or are trying to detect, but to a combination of many other circumstances which we cannot control. An observation is judged significant, if it would rarely have been produced, in the absence of a real cause of the kind we are seeking. It is a common practice to judge a result significant, if it is of such a magnitude that it would have been produced by chance not more frequently than once in twenty trials. This is an *arbitrary, but convenient,* level of significance for the practical investigator, but it does not mean that he allows himself to be deceived once in every twenty experiments. The test of significance only tells him what to ignore, namely all experiments in which significant results are not obtained.
>
> (Salsburg, 2001; p. 99; my italic)

There is no scientific reason for p = 0.05 as opposed to others near it, and here the reader can note that an essential part of the edifice of statistics – this highly mathematical and scientific discipline – has absolutely no basis in science or mathematics at all. Statistics, like all human endeavors, is based, in part, on conceptual assumptions. It is not a science of positive facts through and through.

It is worth pointing out that earlier statisticians in the nineteenth century, though without using the actual phrase "p-value," had developed the concept that the influence of chance needed to be small in making statistical comparisons. How small? Bernoulli used the term "moral certainty" to apply to a likelihood of 1:1000 or less (p < 0.001). Edgeworth suggested a level of certainty equivalent to a p-value of 0.005 (Stigler, 1986). Thus one sees that earlier statisticians suggested a much stricter standard than has become current.

If we appreciate how this 0.05 criterion came about, we might also be more generous and less focused on whether a study result has a p-value of 0.05, or 0.055 (which, God forbid, rounds up to 0.06). I have seen researchers sweat and squirm as a data analysis produces a p-value of 0.06 – the study seems hardly publishable, and certainly less impactful, with that difference of 0.01 from the golden threshold of 0.05.

This is one reason to give less credence to p-values: its cutoff point is arbitrary. But arbitrariness does not imply incoherence. Obviously a p-value above 0.50 (50% chance likelihood) would suggest a truly chance observation. In the lower range of p-values, small differences are not conceptually meaningful. For that reason, we should not treat p-values with reverence – as "mathematical substitutes for sensible thought" – seeking to obtain a magic number almost as if it were a talisman against error, but rather we should interpret p-values for what they are, use them when it makes sense, and refuse to abuse them.

With that context, we should now define what the p-value means. The p stands for probability, and the p-value may be defined as follows: *The probability of observing the observed data, assuming that the null hypothesis (NH) is true.* The p-value is not a real number; it does not reflect a real probability, but rather the likelihood of chance effects *assuming* (but not knowing) that the null condition is true: "It is a theoretical probability associated with observations under conditions that are most likely false. It has nothing to do with reality. It is an indirect measurement of plausibility." (Salsburg, 2001; p. 111.) It is not the probability of an event, but the probability of our *certainty* about an event. Indeed, in this sense, it is a central expression of Laplace's concept of statistics as quantifying, rather than disclaiming, our ignorance (Menand, 2001). A p-value attempts to quantify our ignorance, rather than establish any reality.

Thus, if we use a standard p-value cutoff of 0.05 or less as the definition of *statistical significance,* what we are saying is that *we will be rejecting the NH by mistake 5% of the time or less.*

Note some important misunderstandings:

1. The p-value is *not* the probability of the NH being true.
2. The p-value is *not* the probability of the results occurring *by chance*; it is the probability of the observed results *really* being the case, *if* we assume the NH to be true.

The key relevance for the p-value, as originally developed by Fisher, is not the specific number, but the concept of rareness, the idea that one should examine how likely the play of chance could be, and to interpret one's results more definitively as the likelihood of chance becomes more and more rare. Salsburg notes: "Reading through Fisher's applied papers, one is led to believe that he used significance tests to come to one of three possible conclusions. If the p-value is very small (usually less than .01), he declares that an effect has been shown. If the p-value is large (usually greater than .20), he declares that, if there is an effect, it is so small that no experiment of this size will be able to detect it. If the p-value lies in between, he discusses how the next experiment should be designed to get a better idea of the effect." (Salsburg, 2001; p. 100.)

How p-values led to hypothesis-testing

Originally in the 1920s Fisher developed the p-value concept solely in relation to this notion of statistical significance. Within two decades, however, the use of the p-value and the concept of statistical significance was quickly tied to the concept of rejecting an NH. This evolution occurred through the joint efforts of Fisher's younger colleague Egon Pearson (the son of Fisher's nemesis Karl Pearson) and Jerzy Neyman; hence the hypothesis-testing approach, now standard in mainstream statistics, was originally called the Neyman-Pearson approach.

What Neyman and Pearson faced was the problem that Fisher's p-value seemed to sit in a conceptual void. We knew what it meant if it was very small: the observed results were unlikely to have occurred by chance. But what if a result was non-significant? Does this mean that "a hypothesis is true if we fail to refute it?" (Salsburg, 2001; p. 107.) Recall that Fisher's view was that large p-values would suggest that one could not decide. He clearly stated that a non-significant result does not mean that any hypothesis was thereby proven: we might reject that there *is* a difference, but we have not thereby proven that there is *no* difference. Neyman and Pearson wanted to establish this idea more clearly. They concluded that significance testing with p-values needed to occur in a conceptual structure where two separate alternatives are present: the NH of no difference, and the alternative hypothesis (AH) of a difference. They introduced these now commonplace terms, and, more importantly, the conceptual assumptions upon which our current mega-structure of medical statistics rests. They then defined the probability of detecting the AH as the "power" of a significance test. Now, p-values would not only need to reflect the probability for testing the NH, but they also needed to provide a probability for testing the AH. The concept of power became central as defining a significance test, and false negatives, not just false positives, were better defined (Salsburg, 2001).

Fisher's development of p-values to quantify the probability of chance error in observations led to conceptual problems that Neyman and Pearson tried to solve by devising the concepts of null hypotheses, alternative hypotheses, and power. Fisher was not happy with the additional Neyman-Pearson approach to using p-values, but it has become consecrated now. Called hypothesis-testing, this approach is as central to modern statistics as the supply-and-demand concept is to modern economics. But, just as supply-and-demand economics is at best partially correct, and simply wrong in many ways, so too hypothesis-testing is only sometimes helpful in statistics, and often nothing but a source of confusion and error. Fisher's apprehensions have, frankly, proven true. (It may be relevant that Neyman, who lived into the 1970s, himself rarely used hypothesis-testing methods in his own work; he used confidence intervals, a concept he also originated, much more so, as I will also advocate in Chapter 9.)

The relevance of these debates is that we need to realize that our statistical concepts are not themselves scientific facts, nor did they arrive to us from Mt. Sinai. They are the result of debates which are not yet finished. We need to realize that the above storyline is what happened that led to the first line of most elementary statistics textbooks today. If we don't understand how we got to where we are today, we will misunderstand that first line, and everything that follows.

Definition: what is the null hypothesis?

Since today the definition of the p-value relies on the definition of the NH, let us turn to define the latter.

The NH is an assumption about the nature of the world, required for the use of p-values. The assumption is that things in the world are the same, that they do not differ from each other, and that inductive inferences about relations between things in the world are wrong. Thus stated, we see another assumption at the core of the world of statistics.

In essence, statistics is based on a thought experiment: Let us imagine that nothing of interest was happening in the world. Every time we thought we saw something, every time that we thought some event in the world happened, and every time we thought one thing caused another thing, we would be wrong. The world is unchanging and conservative, always tending toward the negative: things are not happening, observed differences are not real, inferred relationships are wrong. This is the world of the NH. Why should we make this assumption? Why not the opposite assumption? I have not found in the statistical literature a clear conceptual explanation about why the NH is preferable to the opposite thought experiment (the idea, perhaps, that we should accept all differences and relations and inferences that appear to us through induction as real, sometimes called the alternative hypothesis or AH). When comparing the two alternatives, one sees that one is conservative (the NH) and one is liberal (the AH). Why be conservative in science? One argument might be that conservatism is justified in science because we are wrong so often; the history of science might be invoked to show how repeatedly we have been mistaken in our scientific claims. Now that a mathematical method – statistics – has been developed to test scientific theories, it might be rational to use that method to get rid of all the dead wood, all the wrongness, of scientific speculation, as opposed to using statistics to more easily confirm all these ideas and observations that people claim. Another way of putting it, specifically relevant to medical statistics, might be this: Since statistics are influential, once statistics confirm a claim, then doctors and patients are going to be likely to change their practice – they may start using a drug, they may stop using it, they may change their diets, they may start treating children in a certain way, and so on. With these important practical consequences, one might claim that statistics should err on the side of caution, only approving claims when they are highly likely to be true.

This would be a good rationale for the NH, except for the fact that I simply made it up. Not that my invention of it at this time reduces its validity, but it is noteworthy that statisticians themselves have not gone to great lengths to justify the NH as the basis for hypothesis-testing statistics.

When raised, perhaps the classic description is referred to Fisher, who wrote:

> The NH is never proved or established, but is possibly disproved. Every experiment may be said to exist only in order to give the facts a chance of disproving the NH.
>
> (Fisher, 1971 [1935] p. 16)

Thus Fisher admits the essentially speculative character of the NH assumption, and he highlights its central role in the conception of research.

The asymmetry of our concept of the NH is central: we can never prove it; we can perhaps disprove it. Hence, "P is a measure of evidence against the NH, not for it. Insufficient evidence to reject the NH does not imply sufficient evidence to accept it" (Blackwelder, 1982). This problem leads to the need for *non-inferiority* designs as the closest we can get to testing the NH (Chapter 8). We are left with the uncomfortable fact that we cannot empirically (or statistically) test a key concept on which much of statistics rests.

The conservatism assumption

One should be conservative about how to interpret research studies, providing a similar rationale for putting the p-value cutoff at 95% as opposed to 90% or 80%.

Yet there is a cost to this conservatism. Suppose a life-saving treatment arises, but is studied in a sample too small to reach the p-value of 0.05, but instead the treatment leads to a p-value of 0.11. Further, let us suppose that we are God (or gods). We know that this drug is, in fact, quite effective, and let us stipulate that it is much more effective than any other available treatment. Let us also stipulate that it treats a serious illness, and for each year it is not used let us state, being God, that we know that one million persons will die. Now, the statistician, not being God, would only assess the situation this way: First, we assume that the NH is true, that the treatment is ineffective. (Even though God would know this is not true in this case, we mortals always must assume it to be true.) There is an 11% likelihood that the observed treatment effect would have occurred by chance, and thus we have an 11% likelihood that we would incorrectly reject the NH. This 11% possibility of being wrong is too high for us to accept, thus we will continue believing in the NH, i.e., that the treatment is ineffective.

To put it starkly, how many lives are worth a 6% increased risk (11% − 5%) of being wrong by chance? Now this is obviously an extreme situation, and the assumption that we could know the absolute truth like God is obviously false; but the point of thought experiments such as this one, commonly used in academic philosophy, is to bring out our own assumptions, our own intuitions, and their limitations. The problem with the NH approach is that it will automatically be biased (if we wish to use that term, one could also say "weighted") against real findings, real differences, and effective treatments. In cases where such real observations make a major difference in the world, the NH might be too conservative.

One can make this point another way with another thought experiment: Suppose that we are not God, we are mortals, but we know nothing about p-values. We had never heard of them, and we had no awareness of the tradition of a 95% cutoff for chance findings to reject the NH. But we knew all about that terrible illness and its limited available treatments. If I were to tell you, under these circumstances, that this new treatment was extremely effective and that the evidence for this efficacy was 89% *not* likely to be due to chance, would you be inclined to begin using it?

Assumption after assumption

So our first assumption was that p-values should demonstrate that a result was likely to occur outside of chance at the 0.05 level. Our second assumption was that we should accept the NH, and lean toward rejecting observed inferences unless that level of probability of chance findings is shown. These are the two major assumptions of hypothesis-testing methods in statistics. They have some merit, but they also have some weaknesses, and, perhaps most importantly, they are not themselves based on scientific evidence (nor any other stronger form of evidence, such as divine revelation). They are not assumptions that can be, or should be, enforced on humankind as simply right or wrong, but rather they are assumptions, nothing more or nothing less, and if we find them coherent and useful, we can accept them, and if not, we can reject them. Statistics, like any discipline of human knowledge, needs to think about its concepts, instead of rejecting any attempts to question them.

Statistical significance

Now we can examine this term – statistical significance – so widely used in medical research. It basically reflects the p-value cutoff at which the NH can be rejected. Unfortunately, the word "significance" has other uses in the English language outside of statistics, hence this short hand for a statistical result of research is often manipulated for the sometimes less wholesome goals of the human beings who do the research.

Salsburg notes that the original use of the word statistically "significant" by Fisher differs from what it has become: "The word was used in the late-nineteenth-century English meaning, which is simply that the computation *showed or signified something*. As the English language entered the twentieth century, the word *significant* began to take on other meanings, until it developed its current meaning, implying *something very important*." (Salsburg, 2001; p. 98; my italic.) I would emphasize that we need to remember the original meaning of the term: to say that something is statistically significant is to say that *something happened*, e.g., the drug is doing something. It does not mean that *something important happened*, e.g., that the drug is doing something robustly. (The latter connotation of significance requires the use of the effect size concept, see Chapter 9.)

Perhaps the main problem with the concept of statistical significance, however, is that it gives one meaning ("not statistically significant") to a wide range of possible results (p-values ranging from 0.05 to 1.0). Thus, if we only focus on whether a study is statistically significant (SS) or not, then we will say that treatment X with a p-value of 0.07 is not SS and treatment Y with a p-value of 0.94 is also not SS. Yet in one case, the likelihood of a non-chance finding is 93% and in the other case it is 6%. Sometimes researchers use another English word, "trend," to denote those findings that are close to 0.05 but just not quite there (often it is used for p-values between 0.05 and 0.10). Yet when a "statistical trend" is identified, researchers usually are apologetic about it, often feeling the need to explicitly state, in case the reader did not know the statistical meaning of the word "trend," that it is not SS (e.g., "a non-significant trend," or "a statistical trend that is not statistically significant."). I would not be too bothered by the use of the concept of a statistical trend if researchers were able to use the term non-apologetically; but the constant reference to being non-SS undercuts the value of pointing out a statistical trend. The other problem is that this approach only pushes back the problem of the arbitrary cutoff. A p-value of 0.11 is not even a trend, so it is completely meaningless.

In my view, p-values are bad enough; translating p-values into English words with vague meaning ("significance," "trend") is worse. The term SS mostly causes confusion.

Another major problem with the term SS is that it has purely statistical meaning in relation to p-values. It has no meaning in any other way. Yet since the word "significance" in English means, roughly, something that is important, then the words SS tend to be interpreted by doctors and clinicians as meaning, if present, that the results are important, and, if absent, that the results are not important. As will be see in Chapter 8, due to the inherent limitations of p-values, the results of a study may be false positive (and thus the apparently important SS results are in fact not important) or may be false negative (and thus the apparently unimportant SS results are in fact important). Sometimes clinicians try to finesse this problem by talking about "clinical significance" as complementary to SS, using the term clinical significance as a synonym for the more precise term "effect size," which we discuss in Chapter 9. Yet this is uncommonly done, and the continuing multiplication of varieties of "significance" is only bound to lead to more confusion; one is reminded of the interminable quarrels of leftist parties, and their varying definitions of the word "revolution." Perhaps George Orwell had it right: the English language is much more easily abused than used, and we should stick to simple and clear, not vague and abstract, uses of words.

The scope of p-values

There is another feature of p-values that deserves commentary. According to their originator, Ronald Fisher, p-values *should only be used for randomized clinical trials* (RCTs), not for any other kind of scientific research, especially not for observational clinical studies in medicine (Salsburg, 2001; pp. 302–3). This view may seem odd; if true it would invalidate most medical research. But I think Fisher was right, if he is properly understood. The reader will recall the Three C's: the first is confounding bias, the *second* is chance (and the third causation). P-values assess chance; they should not be used unless bias is first removed. Randomized clinical trials remove bias, and thus allow us to skip the first C and move to assessing chance. This was Fisher's insight. Let's give the use of p-values outside of RCTs a name: *Fisher's fallacy*. And this is still where Fisher was correct: if we use p-values willy-nilly, on observational data, without making any effort to reduce confounding or other biases statistically (as with regression models), we are misusing p-values. We cannot assess the minute influence of chance when our data could be massively biased. This was in fact the scientific basis for Fisher's critique of the epidemiological evidence that linked cigarette smoking to lung cancer. If the options are as Fisher had them – either use p-values only in RCTs, or use p-values without further qualification for any kind of study – then Fisher is correct. Where Fisher erred was in not realizing the utility of epidemiological methods to reduce bias in non-RCT settings; regression modeling came later, so Fisher could not have known about it, but these statistical methods allow us to reduce, though not remove, bias, and thus go a long way toward passing the first step of the Three C's and then allowing us to use p-values to assess chance. This was A. Bradford Hill's argument in the cigarette smoking and cancer controversy (see Chapter 10), which laid the foundation of so much of current medical research. One simply cannot do RCTs for every medical matter, and thus epidemiological methods are better than nothing, and provide us more useful knowledge than simply guessing. This is the basic insight behind evidence-based medicine (EBM; see Chapter 12). Fisher could not foresee where this would go, and he did not appreciate the early signs of this approach to valid knowledge outside of RCTs. However, his warning is still an important one: bias comes first, and if it is not removed in some sense (either by RCTs or statistical analyses like regression), then the application of p-values is meaningless. And indeed, most of the psychiatric literature, in particular, still suffers from Fisher's fallacy, and thus misuses p-values.

The faulty logic of hypothesis-testing

There is another important problem with the whole hypothesis-testing approach: it rests on faulty logic. I will briefly make this point here, and then discuss it in more detail in Chapter 11. The prominent statistician Jacob Cohen called it the "illusion of attaining improbability," which is "the widespread belief that the level of significance at which [the NH] is rejected, say .05, is the probability that it is correct or, at the very least, that it is of low probability" (Cohen, 1994). This logic can be described as follows:

> "If the null hypothesis is correct, then these data are highly unlikely.
> These data have occurred.
> Therefore, the null hypothesis is highly unlikely."
>
> (Pollard and Richardson, 1987)

Cohen showed that this logic does not work because it involves probability, which becomes clear once we fill in the abstract data with concrete things:

> If a person is an American then he is probably not a member of Congress. (TRUE, RIGHT?)
> This person is a member of Congress.
> Therefore, he is probably not an American.
>
> (Pollard and Richardson, 1987)

As a senior figure in statistics, and one who put most of his effort into research in psychology, Cohen's reservations, towards the end of his life, have not been sufficiently appreciated:

> We, as teachers, consultants, authors, and otherwise perpetrators of quantitative methods, are responsible for the ritualization of null hypothesis significance testing (NHST; I resisted the temptation to call it statistical hypothesis inference testing) to the point of meaninglessness and beyond. I argue herein that NHST has not only failed to support the advance of psychology as a science but also has seriously impeded it.
>
> (Cohen, 1994)

At a basic level, the faulty probability logic of the NHST leads us astray. At another level, the hypothesis-testing approach sets up a false dichotomy: if the p-value is significant, we accept the hypothesis; if not significant, we reject the hypothesis. This simplistic approach impedes progress in our knowledge, Cohen argues, because science just does not work this way: no single result proves or disproves a scientific hypothesis, but rather, depending on the details of the study, we might be inclined to develop more or less confidence in that hypothesis, based on individual study results. It is far from an all-or-nothing approach to decision-making, but rather a gradual approximation towards or away from a theory (I discuss this philosophy of science further in Chapter 11).

The limits of hypothesis-testing

In sum, the concepts of p-values and statistical significance, though useful when used appropriately, are based on numerous assumptions which are not themselves based on statistics. In other words, there are some important features of these notions that are arbitrary, and open to debate, not simply absolute truths to which we must pledge obedience. Even the formal logic of the hypothesis-testing approach is debatable (see Chapter 11).

This reality should be liberating to clinicians; statistics is not a field in which the numbers alone rule. Just like medicine, just like all human endeavor, statistics involve assumptions and beliefs. So let us not be intimidated by statistics, nor should we devalue it. Unfortunately, most presentations of statistics ignore or whitewash these assumptions that are at the core of the primary axioms of statistics:

> The standard redaction of the Neyman-Pearson formulations found in elementary statistics textbooks tends to present hypothesis testing as a cut-and-dried procedure. Many purely arbitrary aspects of the methods are presented as immutable. While many of these arbitrary elements may not be appropriate for clinical research, the need that some medical scientists have to use 'correct' methods has enshrined an extremely rigid version of the Neyman-Pearson formulation. Nothing is acceptable unless the p-value cutoff is fixed in advance and preserved by the statistical procedure. This was one reason why Fisher opposed the Neyman-Pearson formulation. He did not think that the use of p-values and significance tests should be subjected to such rigorous requirements ... Fisher suggested ... that the final decision about what p-value should be significant should depend upon the circumstances.
>
> (Salsburg, 2001; pp. 278–9)

The use of hypothesis-testing statistics in clinical trials

> It has been rightly observed that while it does not take a great mind to make simple things complicated, it takes a very great mind to make complicated things simple.
>
> Austin Bradford Hill (Hill, 1962; p. 8)

How to design clinical trials

My teachers taught me that when you design a study, the first step is how you plan to analyze it, or how you plan to present the results. One of my teachers even suggested that one should write up the research paper that one would imagine a study would produce – *before conducting the study*. Written of course without the actual numbers, this fantasy exercise has the advantage of pointing out, before a study is designed, exactly what kind of analyses, numbers, and questions need to be answered. The worst thing is to design and complete a study, analyze the data, begin to write the paper, and then realize that an important piece of data was never collected!

Clinical trials: how many questions can we answer?

The clinical trial is how we experiment with human beings. We no longer are dealing with Fisher's different strains of seeds, strewn on differing kinds of soil in a randomized trial. We now have human beings, not seeds, and the resulting clinical trial is how we apply statistical methods of randomization to medical experimentation.

Perhaps the most important feature of clinical trials is that they are designed to answer a single question, but we humans force them to answer hundreds. This is the source of both their power and their debility.

The value of clinical trials comes from this ability to definitively (or as definitively as is possible in this inductive world) answer a single question: does aspirin prevent heart attacks? Does streptomycin cure pneumonia? We want to know these answers. And each single answer, with nothing further said, is worth tons of gold to the health of humankind.

Such a single question is called the *primary outcome* of a clinical trial.

But we researchers and doctors and patients want to know more. Not only do we want to know if aspirin prevents heart attacks, but did it also lead to lower death rates? Did it prevent stroke too perhaps? What kinds of side effects did it cause? Did it cause gastrointestinal bleeding? If so, how many died from such bleeding?

So we seem forced to ask many questions of our clinical trials, partly because we want to know about side effects, but partly just out of our own curiosity: we want to know as much as possible about the effects of a drug on a range of possible benefits.

Sometimes we ask many questions for economic reasons. Clinical trials are expensive; whether a pharmaceutical company or the federal government is paying for it, in either case shareholders or taxpayers will want to get as much as possible out of their investment. You spent $10 million to answer one question? Could you not answer 5 more? Perhaps if you answered 50 questions, the investment would seem even more successful. This may be how it is in business, but in science, the more questions you seek to answer, the fewer you answer well.

False positives and false negatives

The clinical trial is designed primarily to remove the problem of confounding bias, that is, to give us valid data. It removes the problem of bias, but then is faced with the problem of chance.

Chance can lead to false results in two directions, false positives and false negatives.

False positives occur when the p-value is abused. If too many p-values are assessed, then the actual values will be incorrect. An inflation of chance error occurs, and one will be likely to observe many chance positive findings.

False negatives occur when the p-value is abnormally high due to excessive variability in the data. What this means is that there are not enough data points – not enough patients – to limit the variation in the results. The higher the variation, the higher the p-value. Thus, if a study is too small, it will be highly variable in its data, i.e., it will lack precision, and the p-value will be inflated. Thus, the effect will be deemed statistically unworthy.

False positive error is also called *type I or α error*; false negative is called *type II or β error*. The ability to avoid false negative results, by having limited variability and higher precision of the data, is also called *statistical power*.

To avoid both of these kinds of errors, the clinical trial needs to establish a single, primary outcome. By essentially putting all its eggs in one basket, the trial is stating that the p-value for that single analysis should be taken at face value; it will not be distorted by multiple comparisons. Further, by having a primary outcome, the clinical trial can be designed such that a large enough sample size is calculated to limit the variability of the data, improve the precision of the study, and ensure a reasonable likelihood of statistical significance if a certain effect size is obtained.

A clinical trial rises and falls on careful selection of a primary outcome, and careful design of the study and sample size so as to assess the primary outcome.

The primary outcome

The primary outcome is usually some kind of measurement, such as points on a depression rating scale. This measurement can be defined in various ways; for example, it can reflect the actual change in points on a depression rating scale with drug versus placebo; or it can reflect the percentage of responders in drug versus placebo groups (usually defining response as 50% or more improvement in depression rating scale score). In general, the first approach is taken: the actual change in points is compared in the two groups. This is a continuous scale of measurement (1,2,3,4 points …) not a categorical scale (responders versus non-responders), which is a strength. Statistically, continuous measurements provide more data, less variability, and thus more statistical power, thereby enhancing the possibility of a lower p-value. This is the main reason why most primary outcomes in psychiatry and psychology involve continuous rating scale measures.

On the other hand, categorical assessments are often intuitively more understandable by clinicians. Thus, it is typical for a clinical treatment study in psychiatry to be designed mainly to describe a change in depressive symptoms as a number (a continuous change), while also to report the percentage of responders as a second outcome. While both of these outcomes flow one from the other, it is important for researchers to make a choice; they cannot both equally be primary outcomes. A primary outcome is one outcome, and only one outcome. The other is a secondary outcome.

Secondary outcomes

It is natural to want to answer more than one question in a clinical trial. But one needs to be clear which questions are secondary ones, and they need to be distinguished from the primary question. Their results, whether positive or negative, need to be equally interpreted more cautiously than in the case of the primary outcome.

Yet it is not uncommon to see research studies where the primary outcome, such as a continuous change in a depression rating score, may not show a statistically significant benefit, while a secondary outcome, such as categorical response rate, may do so. Researchers then may be tempted to emphasize the categorical response throughout the paper and abstract.

For instance, in a study of risperidone versus placebo added to an antidepressant for treatment-refractory unipolar depression (n = 97) (Keitner et al., 1996), the published abstract reads as follows: "Subjects in both treatment groups improved significantly over time. The odds of remitting were significantly better for patients in the risperidone vs. placebo arm (OR = 3.33, p = .011). At the end of 4 weeks of treatment 52% of the risperidone augmentation group remitted (MADRS10) compared to 24% of the placebo augmentation group (CMH(1) = 6.48, p = .011), but the two groups were converging." Presumably, the continuous mood rating scale scores, which are typically the primary outcome in such randomized clinical trials (RCTs), did not differ between drug and placebo. The abstract is ambiguous. As in this case, often one has trouble identifying any clear statement about which results were the primary outcome and which were secondary outcomes. Without such clarity, one gets the unfortunate result that studies which are negative (on their primary outcomes) are published so as to appear positive (by emphasizing the secondary outcomes).

Not only can secondary outcomes be falsely positive, they can just as commonly be falsely negative. In fact, secondary analyses should be seen as inherently underpowered. An analysis found that, after the single primary outcome, the sample size needed to be about 20% larger for a single secondary outcome, and 30% larger for two secondary outcomes (Leon, 2004).

Post-hoc analyses and subgroup effects

We now reach the vexed problem of subgroup effects. This is the place where, perhaps most directly, statisticians and clinicians have opposite goals. A statistician wants to get results that are as valid as possible and as far removed from chance as possible. This requires isolating one's research question more and more cleanly, such that all other factors can be controlled, and the research question then answered directly. A clinician wants to treat the individual patient, a patient who usually has multiple characteristics (each of us belongs to a certain race, has a certain gender, an age, a social class, a specific history of medical symptoms, and so on), and where the clinical matter at question occurs in the context of those multiple characteristics. The statistician produces an answer for the average patient on an isolated question; the clinician wants an answer for a specific patient with multiple relevant features that influence the clinical question. For the statistician, the question might be: Is antidepressant X better

Table 8.1. Inflation of false positive probabilities with outcomes tested

Number of hypotheses tested	Type I error tested at 0.05 level
1	0.05
2	0.0975
3	0.14
5	0.23
10	0.40
15	0.54
20	0.64
30	0.785
50	0.92
75	0.979
100	0.999

With every hypothesis test at alpha level of 0.05, there is a 1/20 chance the null hypothesis will be rejected by chance. However, to get the probability at least one test would pass if one examines two hypotheses, you cannot multiply 1/20 × 1/20. Instead, one has to multiply the chance the null *would not* be rejected – that is 19/20 × 19/20 (a form of the binomial distribution). Extending this, one can see that the key term would then be 19 n/20 n with n being the number of comparisons, and to get the chance of a Type I error (the null is falsely rejected) the equation would be $1 - 19\,n/20\,n$.

With thanks to Eric G. Smith, MD, MPH (Personal Communication 2008).

than placebo in the average patient? For the clinician, the question might be: Is antidepressant X better than placebo in this specific patient who is African-American, male, 90 years old, with comorbid liver disease? Or, alternatively, is antidepressant X better than placebo in this specific patient who is white, female, 20 years old, with comorbid substance abuse? Neither of them is the "average" patient, if there is such a thing: one would have to imagine a middle-aged person with multiple racial complexity and partial comorbidities of varying kinds.

In other words, if the primary outcome of a clinical trial gives us the "average" result in an "average" patient, how can we apply those results to specific patients? The most common approach, for better and for worse, is to conduct subgroup analyses. In the example above: we might look at the antidepressant response in men versus women, whites versus blacks, old versus young, and so on. Unfortunately, these analyses are usually conducted with p-values, which leads to both false positive and false negative risks, as noted above.

The inflation of p-values

To briefly reiterate, because this matter is worth repeating over and over, the false positive risk is that repeated analyses are a misapplication of the size of the p-value. A p-value of 0.05 means that with one analysis one has a 5% likelihood that the observed result occurred by chance. If ten analyses are conducted, one of which produces a p-value of 0.05, that does NOT mean that the likelihood of that result by chance is 5%; rather it is near 40%. That is the whole concept of a p-value: if analyses are repeated enough, false positive chance findings will occur at a certain frequency, as shown in Table 8.1 in computer simulation by my colleague Eric Smith (personal communication 2008).

Suppose we are willing to accept a p-value of 0.05, meaning that assuming the null hypothesis (NH) is true, the observed difference is likely to occur by chance 5% of the time. The chance of inaccurately accepting a positive finding (rejecting the NH) would be 5% for one comparison, about 10% for two comparisons, 23% for five comparisons, and 40% for ten comparisons. This means that if in an RCT, the primary analysis is negative, but one of four secondary analyses is positive with p = 0.05, then that p-value actually reflects a 23% false positive chance finding, not a 5% false positive chance finding. And we would not accept that higher chance likelihood. Yet clinicians and researchers often do not consider this issue. One option would be to do a correction for multiple comparisons, such as the Bonferroni correction, which would require that the p-value be maintained at 0.05 overall by dividing it by the number of comparisons made. For five comparisons, the acceptable p-value would be 0.05/5, or 0.01. The other approach would be to simply accept the finding, but to give less and less interpretive weight to a positive result as more and more analyses are performed.

This is the main rationale why, when an RCT is designed, researchers should choose one or a few primary outcome measures for which the study should be properly powered (a level of 0.80 or 0.90 [power = 1 − type II error] is a standard convention). Usually there is a main efficacy outcome measure, with one or two secondary efficacy or side effect outcome measures. An efficacy effect or side effect to be tested can be established either a priori (before the study, which is always the case for primary and secondary outcomes) or post hoc (after the fact, which should be viewed as exploratory, not confirmatory, of any hypothesis).

Clinical example: olanzapine prophylaxis of bipolar disorder

In an RCT of olanzapine added to standard mood stabilizers (divalproex or lithium) for prevention of mood episodes in bipolar disorder (Tohen et al., 2004), I have often seen the results presented at conferences as positive, with the combined group of olanzapine plus mood stabilizer preventing relapse better than mood stabilizer alone. But the positive outcome was secondary, not primary. The protocol was designed such that all patients who responded to olanzapine plus divalproex or lithium initially for acute mania would then be randomized to staying on the combination (olanzapine plus mood stabilizer) versus mood stabilizer alone (placebo plus mood stabilizer). The primary outcome was time to a new mood episode (meeting full DSM-IV criteria for mania or depression) in those who responded to olanzapine plus mood stabilizer initially for acute mania (with response defined as > 50% improvement in mania symptom rating scale scores). On this outcome, there was no difference between continuation of olanzapine plus the mood stabilizer or switch to placebo plus mood stabilizer. The primary outcome of this study was negative. Among a number of secondary outcomes, one was positive, defined as time to symptomatic worsening (the recurrence of an increase of manic symptoms or new depressive symptoms, not necessarily full manic or depressive episodes) among those who had initially achieved full remission with olanzapine plus mood stabilizer for acute mania (defined as mania symptom rating scores below 7, i.e., almost no symptoms). On this outcome, the olanzapine plus mood stabilizer combination group had a longer time to symptomatic recurrence than the mood stabilizer alone group (p = 0.023). This p-value does not accurately represent the true chance of a positive finding on this outcome. The published paper does not clearly state how many secondary analyses were conducted a priori, but assuming that one primary analysis was conducted, and two secondary analyses, Table 8.1 indicates that one p-value of 0.05 would be equivalent to a true positive likelihood of 0.14. Thus, the apparent p-value of 0.023 likely represents a true likelihood above the 0.05 usual cutoff for statistical significance. In sum, the positive secondary outcome should be given less weight than the primary outcome because of inflated false positive findings with multiple comparisons.

The astrology of subgroup analysis

One cannot leave this topic without describing a classic study about the false positive risks of subgroup analysis, an analysis which correlated astrological signs with cardiovascular outcomes. In this famous report, the investigators for a well-known study of anti-arrhythmic drugs (ISIS-2) decided to do a subgroup analysis of outcome by astrological sign (Sleight, 2000). (The title of the paper was: "Subgroup analyses in clinical trials: fun to look at – but don't believe them!".) The trial was huge, involving about 17 000 patients, and thus some chance positive findings would be expected with enough analyses in such a large sample. The primary outcome of the study was a comparison of aspirin versus streptokinase for prevention of myocardial infarction, with a finding in favor of aspirin. In subgroup analyses by astrological sign, the authors found that patients born under Gemini or Libra experienced "a slightly adverse effect of aspirin on mortality (9% increase, standard deviation [SD] 13; NS), while for patients born under all other astrological signs there was a striking beneficial effect (28% reduction, SD 5; $p < 0.00001$)."

Either there is something to astrology, or subgroup analyses should be viewed cautiously.

It will not do to think only of positive subgroup results as inherently faulty, however. The false negative risk is just as important; p-values above 0.05 are often called "no difference," when in fact one group can be twice as frequent or larger than the other; yet if the overall frequency of the event is low (as it often is with side effects, see below), then the statistical power of the subgroup analyses will be limited and p-values will be above 0.05. Thinking of how sample size affects statistical power, note that with subgroup analyses samples are being chopped up into smaller groups, and thus statistical power declines notably.

So subgroup analyses are both falsely positive and falsely negative, and yet clinicians will want to ask those questions. Some statisticians recommend holding the line, and refusing to do them. Unfortunately, patients are living people who demand the best answers we can give, even if they are not nearly certain beyond chance likelihood. So let us examine some of the ways statisticians have suggested that the risks of subgroup analyses can be mitigated.

Legitimizing subgroup analyses

Two common approaches follow:

1. Divide the p-value by the number of analyses; this will provide the new level of statistical significance. Called the "Bonferroni correction," the idea is that if ten analyses are conducted, then the standard for significance for any single analysis would be $0.05/10 = 0.005$. The higher threshold of 0.5%, rather than 5%, would be used to call a result unlikely to have happened by chance. This approach draws the p-value noose as tightly as possible, so that what passes through is likely true, but much that is true fails to pass through. Some more liberal alternatives (such as the Tukey test) exist, but all such approaches are guesses about levels of significance, which can be either too conservative or too liberal.

2. Choose the subgroup analyses before the study, a priori, rather than post hoc. The problem with post-hoc analyses is that, almost always, researchers do not report how many such

analyses were conducted. Thus, if a report states that subgroup analysis X found a p = 0.04, we do not know if it was one of only 5, or one of 500, analyses conducted. As noted above, there is a huge difference in how we would interpret that p-value depending on the denominator of how many times it was tested in different subgroup analyses. By stating a priori, before any data analysis occurs, that we plan to conduct a subgroup analysis, that suspicion is removed for readers. However, if one states that one plans to do 25 a-priori subgroup analyses, those are still subject to the same inflation of p-value false positive findings as noted above.

In the *New England Journal of Medicine*, the most widely-read medical journal, which is generally seen as having among the highest statistical standards, a recent review of 95 RCTs published there found that 61% conducted subgroup analyses (Wang *et al.*, 2007). Of these RCTs with subgroup analyses, 43% were not clear about whether the analyses were a priori or post hoc, and 67% conducted five or more subgroup analyses. Thus, even in the strictest medical journals, about half of subgroup analyses are not reported clearly or conducted conservatively.

Some authors also point out that subgroup analyses are weakened by the fact that they generally examine features that may influence results one by one. Thus drug response is compared by gender, then by race, then by social class, and so on. This is equivalent, as described previously (see Chapter 6), to univariate statistical comparisons as opposed to multivariate analyses. The problem is that women may not differ from men in drug response, but perhaps white women differ from African-American men, or perhaps white older women differ from African-American younger men. In other words, multiple clinical features may go together, and, as a group but not singly, influence the outcome. These possibilities are not captured in typical subgroup effect analyses. Some authors recommend, therefore, that after an RCT is complete, multivariate regression models be conducted in search of possible subgroup effects (Kent and Hayward, 2007). Again, while clinically relevant, this approach still will have notable false positive and false negative risks.

In sum, clinical trials do well in answering the primary question which they are designed to answer. Further questions can only be answered with decreasing levels of confidence with standard hypothesis-testing statistics. As described later, I will advocate that these limitations make the use of hypothesis-testing statistics irrelevant, and that we should turn to descriptive statistical methods instead in looking at clinical subgroups in RCTs.

Power analysis

Most authors focus on the false positive risks of subgroup analyses. But important false negative risks also exist. This brings us to the question of statistical power. We might define this term as the ability of the study to identify the result in question; to put it another way, how likely is the study to note that a difference between two groups is statistically significant? Power depends on three factors, two of which are sample size and variability of data. Most authors focus on sample size, but data variability is just as relevant. In fact, the two factors go together: the larger the sample, the smaller the data variability; the smaller the sample, the larger the data variability. The benefit of large samples is that, as more and more subjects are included in a study, the results become more and more consistent: everybody tends towards getting the same result; hence there is less variability in the data. The typical measure of the variability of the data is the SD.

The third factor, also frequently ignored, is the effect size: the larger the effect size, the greater the power of the study; the smaller the effect size, the lower the statistical power. Sometimes, an effect of a treatment might be so strong and so definitive, however, that even with a small sample, the study subjects tend to consistently get the same result, and thus the data variability is also small. In that example, statistical power will be rather good even though the sample size is small, as long as there is a large effect size and a low SD.

In contrast, a highly underpowered study will have a small effect size, high data variability (large SD), and a small sample size. We often face this latter circumstance in the scenario of medication side effects (see below).

The equation used to calculate statistical power reflects the relationships between these three variables:

Statistical power (or β, see below) = Effect size × sample size/standard deviation.

Thus, the larger the numerator (large sample, large effect size) or the smaller the denominator (small SD), the larger the statistical power.

The mathematical notation used for statistical power is "β," with β error reflecting the false negative risk (just as "α" error reflecting the false positive risk, i.e., the p-value as discussed previously). Beta reflects the probability of not rejecting the alternative hypothesis (AH; the idea that the NH is false, i.e., a real difference exists in a study) when the AH is true. The contrast with the p-value or α error is that α is the probability of rejecting the NH when the NH is true.

As discussed previously, the somewhat arbitrary standard for false positive risk, or α error, is 5% (p or α = 0.05). We are willing to mistakenly reject the NH up to the point where the data are 95% or more certain to be free from chance occurrence. The equally arbitrary standard for β error is 80% (β = 0.80): we are willing to mistakenly reject the AH up to the point where the data are 80% or more certain to be free from chance occurrence. Note that standard statistical practice is to be willing to risk false negatives 20% of the time, but false positives only 5% of the time: in other words, a higher threshold is placed on saying that a real difference exists in the data (rejecting the NH) than is placed on saying that no real difference exists in the data (rejecting the AH). This is another way of saying that statistical standards are biased towards more false negative findings than false positive findings. Why? There is no real reason.

One might speculate, in the case of medical statistics, that it matters more if we are wrong when we say that differences exist (e.g., that treatments work) than when we say that no differences exist (e.g., that treatments do not work), because treatments can cause harm (side effects).

The subjectivity of power analysis

Although many statisticians have made a fuss about the need to conduct power analyses, noting that many research studies are not sufficiently powered to assess their outcomes, in practice power analysis can be a rather subjective affair, a kind of quantitative hand-waving. For instance, suppose I want to show that drug X will be better than placebo by a 25% difference in a depression rating scale. Using standard power calculations, I need to know two things to determine my needed sample size: the hypothesized difference between drug and placebo (the effect size), and the expected SD (the variability of the data). For an acceptable power estimate of 80% (for β), and an expected effect size of 25% difference between drug and placebo, one gets quite differing results depending on how one estimates the SD. Here one needs to convert estimates to absolute numbers: suppose the depression rating scale improvement was expected to be 10 points with drug; 25% difference would mean that placebo would lead to a 7.5 point improvement. The mean difference between the two groups would be 2.5 points (10 − 7.5). Standard deviation is commonly assessed as follows: If it is equal to the actual mean, then there is notable (but acceptable) variability; if it is smaller than the actual mean, then there is not much variability; if it is larger than the actual mean, then there is excessive variability. Thus, if we use a mean change of 7.5 points in the drug group as our standard, a good SD would be about 5 (not much variability, most patients responded similarly), acceptable but bothersome would be 7.5, and too much variability would be an SD of 10 or more. Using these different SDs in our power analysis produces rather different results (internet-based sample size calculators can easily be used for these calculations; I used http://www.stat.ubc.ca/~rollin/stats/ssize/n2.html, accessed August 22, 2008): with low SD = 5, the above power analysis produces a needed sample size of 126; with medium SD = 7.5, the sample needed would be 284; and with high SD = 10, the sample needed would jump massively to 504. Which should we pick? As a researcher perhaps with limited resources or trying to convince an agency or company to fund my study, I would try to produce the lowest number, and I could do so by claiming a low SD. Do I really know beforehand that the study will produce low variability in the data? No. It might; it might not. It may turn out that patients respond quite differently, and if the SD is large, then my study will turn out to be underpowered. One might deal with this problem by routinely picking a middle-range SD, like 7.5 in this example; but few researchers actually plan for the worst case scenario, with a large SD, which would make many studies infeasibly large and in some cases overpowered (if the study turns out to have less variability than in the worst case scenario).

The point of this example is to show that there are many assumptions that go into power analysis, based on guesswork, and that the process is not simply based on "facts" or hard data.

Side effects

As a corollary of the need to limit the number of p-values, a common error in assessing the results of a clinical trial or of an observational study is to evaluate side effects across patient groups based on whether or not they differ on p-values (e.g., drug vs. placebo group). However, most clinical studies are not powered to assess side effects, especially when side effects are not frequent. Significance testing is not appropriate, since the risk of a false negative finding using this technique in isolation is too high.

Side effects should not be interpreted based on p-values and significance testing because of the high false negative (type II) error risk. They are not hypotheses to be tested, but simply observations to be reported. The appropriate statistical approach is to report the effect size (e.g., percent) with 95% confidence intervals (CIs; the range of expected estimated observations based on repeated studies).

These issues are directly relevant to the question of whether a drug has a risk of causing mania. In the case of lamotrigine, for instance, a review of the pooled clinical trials failed to find a difference with placebo (Table 8.2).

Those studies were not designed to detect such a difference. It may indeed be that lamotrigine is not higher risk than placebo, but it is concerning that the overall risk of pure manic episodes (1.3%) is fourfold higher than placebo (0.3%) (relative risk = 4.14, 95%

Table 8.2. Treatment-emergent mood events: all controlled studies to date

	Lamotrigine* (n = 379)	Placebo** (n = 314)	Test Statistic	Relative Risk	95% Confidence Intervals
Hypomania	2.1%	1.9%	$x^2 = 0.01, p = 0.93$	1.10	0.39–3.15
Mania	1.3%	0.3%	$x^2 = 1.01, p = 0.32$	4.14	0.49–35.27
Mixed Episode	0.3%	0.3%	$x^2 = 0.33, p = 0.56$	0.83	0.05–13.19
All events	3.7%	2.5%	$x^2 = 0.41, p = 0.52$	1.45	0.62–3.41

* Bipolar disorder, n = 232, Unipolar disorder, n = 147
** Bipolar disorder, n = 166, Unipolar disorder, n = 148
From Ghaemi, S. N. *et al.* (2003) with permission.

CI 0.49–35.27): in fact, the sample size required to "statistically" detect (i.e., using "significance hypothesis-testing" procedures) this observed difference in pure mania would be achieved with a study comparing two arms of almost 1500 patients each (at a type II error level of 0.80, with statistical assumptions of no dropouts, perfect compliance, and equal-sized arms).

To give another example, if we accept a spontaneous baseline manic-switch rate of about 5% over two months of observation, and further assume that the minimal "clinically" relevant difference to be detected is a doubling of all events at a 10% rate in the lamotrigine group, the required sample size of a study properly powered to "statistically" detect this "clinically" significant difference should be almost 1000 overall (assuming no dropouts, perfect compliance and equal-sized arms). Only with such a sample we could be confident that a reported p-value greater than 0.05 really reflects a substantial, clinical equivalence of lamotrigine and placebo in causing acute mania. These pooled data involved 693 patients, which is somewhat more than half the needed sample, but even larger samples would be needed due to the statistical assumptions requiring no dropouts, full compliance, and equal sample size in both arms.

The methodological point is that one cannot assume no difference when studies are not designed to test a hypothesis.

The problem of dropouts and intent to treat (ITT) analysis

Even if patients agree to participate in RCTs, one cannot expect that they will remain in those studies until the end. Humans are humans, and they may change their minds, or they might move away, or they might just get tired of coming to appointments; they could also have side effects or stop treatment because they are not getting better. Whatever the cause, when patients cannot complete an RCT, major problems arise in interpreting the results. The solution to the problem is usually the use of intent to treat (ITT) analyses.

What this means is that randomization equalizes all potential confounding factors for the entire sample at the beginning of the study. If that entire sample is analyzed at the end of the study, there should be no confounding bias. However, if some of that sample is not analyzed at the end of the study (as in completer analysis where dropouts before the end of the study are not analyzed), then one cannot be sure that the two groups at the end of the study are still equal on all potential confounding factors. If some patients drop out of one treatment arm because of less efficacy, or more side effects, then these non-random dropouts will bias the ultimate results of the study in a completer analysis. Thus, in general, an ITT approach is used. From the study design perspective, this is called ITT because we intend to treat all the patients for the entire duration of the study, whether or not they stay in the study until the very end. From the statistical analysis perspective, ITT is related to the last observation carried forward (LOCF) approach because it comes down to taking the last data point available for the patient and pretending that it occurred at the very end of the study. The problem with this approach is that it obviously assumes that the last outcome for the patient in the study would have remained the same until the very end of the study, i.e., that the patient would not have gotten any better or any worse. This is less of a problem in a short-term as opposed to a maintenance study. Nonetheless, it is important to realize that there are assumptions built into both LOCF and completer analyses and that none of them fully remove all possibility of bias.

Intent to treat analysis, like so much of statistics (and most of life), is not perfect, but it is the best approach we have: it minimizes bias more than other approaches. It is a means to deal with the fact that humans are not animals, and that RCTs cannot possibly lead to absolute environmental control. We may randomize patients to a treatment, but, unless we wish to go Stalinist, we cannot force them to remain on that treatment. The statistician who developed it, Richard Peto, realized its limitations fully while also realizing its value. As summarized by Salsburg: "This approach may seem foolish at first glance. One can produce scenarios in which a standard treatment is being compared to an experimental one, with patients switched to the standard if they fail. Then, if the experimental treatment is worthless, all or most of the patients randomized to it will be switched to the standard, and the analysis will find the two treatments the same. As Richard Peto made it clear in his proposal, this method of analyzing the results of a study cannot be used to find that treatments are equivalent. It can only be used if the analysis finds that they *differ* in effect." (Salsburg, 2001; p. 277.) In other words, the residual bias with ITT analysis should work *against* benefit with an experimental drug, and thus any benefit seen in an ITT analysis is not likely to have been inflated.

The presence of some potential for bias in even the best crafted RCT means that one can never be completely certain that the results of any RCT are valid. This raises the need for replication with multiple RCTs to get closer to establishing causation.

Generalizability

A cost to the above efforts to conduct clinical trials efficiently is that one can enhance the study validity at the expense of generalizability: some use the terms internal versus external validity to make the same point.

After crossing the hurdles of confounding bias and chance, a reader might conclude that the results of a study are valid. The final step is to assess the scope of these valid results. We then move to the topic of generalizability, which is quite different than validity. For generalizability (sometimes called external validity, as opposed to internal validity), one should ask the question: given that these results are right, to whom do they apply? In other words, who was in the sample? More directly, clinicians might want to compare their own patients to those in the sample to determine which of their patients might be affected by what they learned from that study. To some extent, validity is a relative concept: e.g., investigators observe that one group of patients does better than another. But generalizability is an absolute concept: how many patients did better? And who were those patients? One has to search the methods section carefully to answer this question, usually by looking for the "inclusion and exclusion criteria" of a study.

One way in which generalizability is discussed is often by using the term *efficacy* for the results of the samples of patients in clinical trials, and *effectiveness* for the results in larger populations of patients in the real-world. "Services research" has developed as a field partly to emphasize the need for generalizable data obtained from non-clinical trial populations.

If patients have to go through all the hoops of randomization, and blinding, and placebo, and rating scales, and so on, one might expect that only some patients would agree to participate in research studies with all those limitations. Some studies found that the simple use of placebo automatically excludes many patients: about one-half of patients with schizophrenia stated that they would refuse to participate in any study simply if it used placebo (Roberts *et al.*, 2002; Hummer *et al.*, 2003). Once one adds other demands of research (acceptance of randomization, frequent visits, blinding), one can expect that the majority of patients with major mental illnesses would refuse to participate in most RCTs. Then when one adds the fact that there are always exclusion criteria, sometimes stringent, to all studies (often, for instance, exclusion of those with active substance abuse, or those who are non-compliant with appointments), then one may get the sense of how the RCT literature, which provides the most valid data and is the basis for most of treatment decisions, is drawn from a small sliver of patients from the larger pie of persons with illnesses. One study of elderly depression found that only 4.2% of 188 severely depressed elderly patients were able to enter an antidepressant study (mostly due to exclusion due to concomitant psychiatric or medical illnesses) (Yastrubetskaya *et al.*, 1997). Another research group applied standard exclusion criteria in many antidepressant clinical trials (mainly psychiatric and substance abuse comorbidities or current suicidal ideation) to 293 patients who they had diagnosed with a unipolar current major depressive episode in regular clinical practice (Zimmerman *et al.*, 2002). They found that only 14% of patients would have met standard inclusion criteria for antidepressant clinical trials. Assuming that about one-half or so would simply refuse to take placebo or receive blinded treatment, one can estimate that less than 10% would ultimately have participated in antidepressant RCTs.

Perhaps that number is a valid estimate: for any major psychiatric condition, about 10% of patients with the relevant diagnosis will qualify for and agree to participate in available RCTs. The assumption in the world of clinical trials is that the research conducted on this 10% is generalizable to the other 90%. This may or may not be the case, and there is no clear way to prove or disprove the matter. It is just another place where statistics has its limits, and where clinicians should use statistical data with judgment (not simply rejecting nor unthinkingly accepting them).

Clinical example: maintenance studies of bipolar disorder

Generalizability is a major issue in certain settings. A good example is maintenance studies of bipolar disorder, where there are two basic study designs: prophylaxis and relapse prevention. In the prophylaxis design, "all comers" are included in the study: in other words, any patient who is euthymic, no matter how that person got well, is eligible to be randomized to drug versus placebo or control. In the relapse prevention design, only those patients who acutely respond to the drug being studied are then eligible to enter the maintenance phase, which is when the study begins. Those who responded to the drug are then randomized to stay on the drug or be switched to placebo or control. These are obviously not testing the same kinds of patients.

Here is a clinical example: The only divalproex maintenance study (Bowden *et al.*, 2000), which used the prophylaxis design, failed to find a difference between that agent, lithium, and placebo. Part of the reason for that failure has been attributed to the prophylaxis design, which may inflate placebo rates. For instance, if someone was euthymic for ten years due to natural history, that person could enter a prophylaxis design and if assigned to placebo, might remain euthymic for years to come due to a natural history of very long periods of wellness. On the other hand, the relapse prevention design enhances the effect size for the study drug, since those who remain on it have already been selected to be good responders to it. In a secondary analysis of the divalproex maintenance study, those who initially responded to divalproex before entering the study (relapse prevention design) had better outcomes with divalproex compared to placebo. This analysis was not definitive, however, because it was a secondary analysis. In contrast, later studies (Gyulai *et al.*, 2003) with lamotrigine and olanzapine all used relapse prevention designs: only responders to lamotrigine or olanzapine entered those studies. Thus, the positive results of those studies do not indicate greater efficacy than divalproex, given the differences in design.

A problem with the relapse prevention design is that it introduces the possibility of a withdrawal syndrome. Those treated with placebo are in fact persons who responded acutely to the study drug *for a certain amount of time*, and then get discontinued, often abruptly. This kind of outcome may be relevant to a recent maintenance study of olanzapine versus placebo, in which all patients who entered the study initially had to be open responder to olanzapine for acute mania *for a minimum of two weeks* (Tohen *et al.*, 2000). In that study, the placebo relapse rate was very high and almost exclusively limited to the first 1–2 months after study initiation, which may represent withdrawal relapse after recent acute efficacy. Almost the entire difference between olanzapine and placebo had to do with relapse within 2 months after recovery from the acute episode. This represents continuation, not maintenance, phase efficacy, which I would define as 6 months or longer (Ghaemi, 2007).

In many recent maintenance relapse prevention studies of lamotrigine, lithium is included as an active control. Since the study is not designed and powered to assess lithium efficacy, definitive conclusions about lithium's efficacy cannot be made from these studies. Further, since the sample is enriched to select lamotrigine responders, it is not an equal comparison of lithium and lamotrigine in an unselected sample. It is really a comparison of how lamotrigine responders might respond to being put on lithium for maintenance, rather than continuing lamotrigine. Thus, it does not necessarily follow from these studies that lamotrigine is more effective than lithium in prevention of depressive episodes (one of the frequently emphasized secondary outcomes) (Goodwin *et al.*, 2004).

Another example of the issue of generalizability involves studies of combination therapy, often with an atypical antipsychotic plus a standard mood stabilizer, versus mood stabilizer monotherapy in treatment of acute mania. Those studies tend to routinely show benefit with combination treatment, yet it is important to note that the majority of patients in those studies initially must fail to respond to mood stabilizer monotherapy. Thus, the comparison is between an already failed treatment (mood stabilizer monotherapy) versus a new treatment (combination treatment). In one study (Sachs *et al.*, 2002) of risperidone in mania, about one-third of the sample had not been previously treated with mood stabilizer, and thus were not selected for mood stabilizer non-response. Those patients entered the study initially without any treatment. They were then randomized to mood stabilizer alone (lithium or valproate or carbamazepine based on patient/doctor preference) versus mood stabilizer plus risperidone. Much less benefit with risperidone was seen when patients were not preselected for having already failed mood stabilizer monotherapy. In sum, such studies which tend to support combination therapy with antipsychotic plus mood stabilizer are likely only generalizable to those who have failed mood stabilizer monotherapy. One *cannot* conclude, as is often heard, that combination therapy with these two classes of drugs is *generally* more effective than mood stabilizers alone.

The need for balance

Here is another place where numbers do not stand alone, another example of where we need to use concepts in statistics, rather than simply calculations. Sampling from the larger population is unavoidable; thus one must accept the results of samples while also paying attention to any unique features that may make them less generalizable. A balance is required: "Since the investigator can describe only to a limited extent the kinds of participants in whom an intervention was evaluated, a *leap of faith* is always required when applying any study findings to the population with the condition. In taking this jump, one must always strike a balance between making unjustifiably broad generalizations and being too conservative in one's claims" (Friedman *et al.*, 1998; p. 38; my italic).

Placebo

Many think that placebos are the most important aspect of clinical trials. This view is mistaken. Rather, as should be clear by now, randomization is the most important feature. Placebos usually go along with blinding, though some double-blind trials employ drugs only, without placebo. Many randomized studies, however, are perfectly valid without the use of any placebo. Thus, placebos are not the *sine qua non* of clinical trials: randomization is.

The principle rationale for using placebo is to control for the natural history of the illness. It is not because there are no active treatments available, and it is not because we want to maximize the drug-related effect size, though those features matter. The most important thing is to realize that most psychiatric illnesses resolve spontaneously, at least short-term, and thus placebo is needed to show that the use of drugs is associated with enough benefit over the natural history to outweigh the risks.

A common misconception is that benefits with placebo involve an inherent "placebo effect," which may consist of non-specific psychosocial supportive factors, or possibly specific biological effects (Shepherd, 1993). Such discussions often forget the effect of Nature (or God if one prefers): the natural healing process. It is this natural history which is the essence of the placebo effect, although it might be augmented by non-specific psychosocial supportive factors as well.

It is not even clear that the placebo effect is much of an effect, though many non-researchers, especially psychotherapists, often assume that the placebo effect involves some relationship to supportive psychotherapy. A recent review of RCTs which had a placebo arm and a no treatment arm – i.e., some patients who did not receive a placebo pill and also were not treated at all – found that placebo was not more effective than no treatment (Hrobjartsson and Gotzsche, 2001).

Thus, many of our assumptions regarding placebo effects may need to be viewed as preliminary. I suggest that the main claim that can be best supported for now is that placebos reflect the natural history of the untreated illness.

In applying this discussion to RCTs of antidepressants, a recent large meta-analysis of the Food and Drug Administration (FDA) database (which includes negative unpublished studies, see Chapter 17) argued that the benefits of drug over placebo involve a very small effect size, when all RCTs are pooled in meta-analysis (Kirsch *et al.*, 2008). One should keep in mind though that meta-analysis (see Chapter 13), by pooling different studies, mixes apples and oranges, and a straightforward interpretation of the data, as with RCTs, is no longer valid. Rather, some of those RCTs involved mildly depressed subjects; others more severely depressed subjects. Pooling them together does not allow one to validly generalize to those who are severely depressed, for instance. When looking at the severely depressed population, it appears that there is a larger beneficial effect size of antidepressants over placebo, mainly because of a lower placebo response in those patients (Kirsch *et al.*, 2008), likely reflecting a more severe natural history of illness.

Many critics think that placebos should *never* be used when a proven active treatment is available, viewing it as unethical to withhold such treatment. The main argument against always comparing new drugs to active proven treatments (Moncrieff *et al.*, 1998) is that the effect size will be smaller between those two groups, and thus larger numbers of people will be exposed to potentially ineffective or harmful drugs in RCTs. If fewer people can be studied with RCTs when placebo is used, and a drug turns out to be ineffective or harmful, then fewer people are exposed to risk (Emanuel and Miller, 2001).

Summary

Randomized clinical trials have revolutionized medicine, yet they have many limitations. This is a reason not to view them as sufficient unto themselves, as in ivory-tower evidence-based medicine, but it is not a reason to devalue them as unnecessary (see Chapter 12). Once again, the most important tool is knowledge, so that RCTs can be adequately evaluated, and the important knowledge that clinicians need is drawn from them, while mistaken interpretations are avoided.

The better alternative: effect estimation

It is better to have an approximate answer to the right question than an exact answer to the wrong one.

John Tukey (Salsburg, 2001; p. 231)

One should not get too fancy with statistics. Most of the time, the best statistics are simply descriptive, often called effect estimation.

The effect estimation approach breaks out the factors of effect size and precision (or variability of the data), and provides more information, and in a more clearly presented form, than the hypothesis-testing approach. The main advantage of the effect estimation approach is that it does not require a pre-existing hypothesis (such as the null and alternative hypotheses), and thus we do not get into all the hazards of false negative and false positive results.

The best way to understand effect estimation, the alternative to hypothesis-testing, is to appreciate the classic concept of a 2 × 2 table (Table 9.1). Here you have two groups: one that had the exposure (or treatment) and one that did not. Then you have two outcomes: yes or no (response or non-response; illness or non-illness).

Using a drug treatment for depression as an example, the effect size can simply be the percentage of responders: number who responded (a + c) ÷ number treated (a + b). Or it can be a relative risk: the likelihood of responding if given treatment would be a/a + b; the likelihood of responding if not given treatment would be c/c + d. So the relative likelihood of responding if given the treatment would be a/a + b ÷ c/c + d. This is often called the risk ratio and abbreviated as RR.

Another measure of relative risk is the odds ratio, abbreviated as OR, which mathematically equals ad/bc. The OR is related to, but not the same as, the RR. Odds are used to estimate probabilities, most commonly in settings of gambling. Probabilities can be said to range from 0% likelihood to 50−50 (meaning chance likelihood in either direction) to 100% absolute likelihood. Odds are defined as p/1 − p if p is the probability of an event. Thus if the probability is 50% (or colloquially "50–50"), then the odds are 0.5/1 − 0.5 = 1. This is often expressed as "1 to 1." If the probability is absolutely likely, meaning 100%, then the odds are infinite: 1/1 − 1 = 1/0 = Infinity. Odds ratios approximate RRs; the only reason to distinguish them is that ORs are mathematically useful in regression models. When not using regression models, RRs are more intuitively straightforward.

The effect size

The effect estimation approach to statistics thus involves using effect sizes, such as relative risks, as the main number of interest. The *effect size*, or the actual estimate of effect, is a number; this is whatever the number is: it may be a percentage (68% of patients were responders),

Table 9.1. The epidemiological two-by-two table

	Outcome: yes	Outcome: no	
Exposure: yes	a	b	a + b
Exposure: no	c	d	c + d
	a + c	b + d	

or an actual number (the mean depression rating scale score was 12.4), or, quite commonly, a relative risk estimate: risk ratios (RRs) or odds ratios (ORs).

Many people use the word effect size to mean *standardized effect size*, which is a special kind of effect estimate. The standardized effect size, called *Cohen's d*, is the actual effect size described above (such as a mean number) divided by the standard deviation (the measure of variability). It produces a number that ranges from 0 to 1 or higher, and these numbers have meaning, but not unless one is familiar with the concept. Generally, it is said that a Cohen's d effect size of 0.4 or lower is small, 0.4 to 0.7 medium, and above 0.7 large. Cohen's d is a useful measure of effect because it corrects for the variability of the sample, but it is less interpretable sometimes than the actual unadulterated effect size. For instance, if we report that the mean Hamilton depression rating scale score (usually above 20 for severe depression) was 0.5 (zero being no symptoms) after treatment, we can know that the effect size is large, without needing to divide it by the standard deviation and get a Cohen's d greater than 1. Nonetheless, Cohen's d is especially useful in research using continuous measures of outcome (such as psychiatric rating scales) and is commonly employed in experimental psychology research.

Other important estimates of effect, newer and more relevant to clinical psychiatry, is the *number needed to treat* (NNT) and the *number needed to harm* (NNH). This is a way of trying to give the effect estimate in a clinically meaningful way. Let us suppose that 60% of patients responded to a drug and 40% to placebo. One way to express the effect size is the RR of 1.5 (60% divided by 40%). Another way of looking at it is that the difference between the two groups is 20% (60% − 40%). This is called the absolute risk reduction (ARR). The NNT is the reciprocal of the ARR, or 1/ARR, in this case 1/0.20 = 5. Thus, for this kind of 20% difference between drug and placebo, clinically we can conclude that we need to treat five patients with the drug to get benefit in one of them. Again, certain standards are needed. Generally, it is viewed that an NNT of 5 or less is very large, 5–10 is large, 10–20 is moderate, above 20 is small, and above 50 is very small.

A note of caution: this kind of abstract categorization of the size of the NNT is not exactly accurate. The NNT by itself may not fully capture whether an effect size is large or small. Some authors (Kraemer and Kupfer, 2006) note, for instance, that the NNT for prevention of heart attack with aspirin is 130; the NNT for cyclosporine prevention of organ rejection is 6.3; and the NNT for effectiveness of psychotherapy (based on one review of the literature) is 3.1 Yet aspirin is widely recommended, cyclosporine is seen as a breakthrough, and psychotherapy is seen as "modest" in benefit. The explanation for these interpretations might be that the "hard" outcome of heart attack may justify a larger NNT with aspirin, as opposed to the "soft" outcome of feeling better after psychotherapy. Aspirin is also cheap and easy to obtain, while psychotherapy is expensive and time-consuming (similarly, cyclosporine is expensive and associated with many medical risks).

Number needed to treat provides effect sizes, therefore, which need to be interpreted in the setting of the outcome being prevented and the costs and risks of the treatment being given.

The converse of the NNT is the NNH, which is used when assessing side effects. Similar considerations apply to NNH, and it is calculated in a similar way as the NNT. Thus, if an antipsychotic drug causes akathisia in 20% of patients versus 5% with placebo, then the ARR is 15% (20% − 5%), and the NNH is $1/0.15 = 6.7$.

The meaning of confidence intervals

Jerzy Neyman, who developed the basic structure of hypothesis-testing statistics (Chapter 7), also advanced the alternative approach of effect estimation with the concept of *confidence intervals* (CIs) (in 1934).

The rationale for CIs stems from the fact that we are dealing with probabilities in statistics and in all medical research. We observe something, say a 45.9% response rate with drug Y. Is the real value 45.9%; not 45.6%, or 46.3%? How much *confidence* do we have in the number we observe? In traditional statistics, the view is that there is a real number that we are trying to discover (let's say that God, who knows all, knows that the real response rate with drug Y is 46.1%). Our observed number is a *statistic*, an estimate of the real number. (Fisher had defined the word statistic "as a number that is derived from the observed measurements and that estimates a parameter of the distribution." (Salsburg, 2001; p. 89).) But we need to have some sense of how plausible our statistic is, how well it reflects the likely real number. The concept of CIs as developed by Neyman was not itself a probability; this was not just another variation of p-values. Rather Neyman saw it as a conceptual construct that helped us appreciate how well our observations have approached reality. As Salsburg puts it: "the confidence interval has to be viewed not in terms of each conclusion but as a process. In the long run, the statistician who always computes 95 percent confidence intervals will find that the true value of the parameter lies within the computed interval 95 percent of the time. Note that, to Neyman, the probability associated with the confidence interval was not the probability that we are correct. It was the frequency of correct statements that a statistician who uses his method will make in the long run. It says nothing about how 'accurate' the current estimate is." (Salsburg, 2001; p. 123.)

We can, therefore, make the following statements: *CIs* can be defined as *the range of plausible values* for the effect size. Another way of putting it is that it is *the likelihood that the real value for the variable would be captured in 95% of trials*. Or, alternatively, *if the study was repeated over and over again, the observed results would fall within the CIs 95% of the time*. (More formally defined, the CI is: "The interval computed from sample data that has a given probability that the unknown parameter ... is contained within the interval." (Dawson and Trapp, 2001; p. 335.)

Confidence intervals use a theoretical computation that involves the mean and the standard deviation, or variability, of the distribution. This can be stated as follows: The CI for a mean is the "Observed mean ± (confidence coefficient) × Variability of the mean" (Dawson and Trapp, 2001). The CI uses mathematical formulae similar to what are used to calculate p-values (each extreme is computed at 1.96 standard deviations from the mean in a normal distribution), and thus the 95% limit of a CI is equivalent to a p-value = 0.05. This is why CIs can give the same information as p-values, but CIs also give much more: the probability of the observed findings when compared to that computed normal distribution.

The CI is *not* the probability of detecting the true parameter. It does not mean that you have a 95% probability of having detected the true value of the variable. The true value has

Table 9.2. American College of Neuropsychopharmacology (ACNP) review of risk of suicidality with antidepressants

Medication	n	Suicide deaths	Percent of youth with suicidal behavior or ideation		P value	Statistical significance
			Antidepressant	Placebo		
Citalopram	418	0	8.9%	7.3%	0.5	Not significant
Fluoxetine	458	0	3.6%	3.8%	0.9	Not significant
Paroxetine	669	0	3.7%	2.5%	0.4	Not significant
Sertraline	376	0	2.7%	1.1%	0.3	Not significant
Venlafaxine	334	0	2.0%	0%	0.25	Not significant
		Total:	2.40%	1.42%	RR = 1.65	95% CI [1.07, 2.55]

The ACNP report did not provide the final line summarizing the total percentages and providing RR and CIs, which I calculated.
From American College of Neuropsychopharmacology (2004) with permission from ACNP.

either been detected or not; we do not know whether it has fallen within our CIs. The CIs instead reflect the likelihood of such being the case with repeated testing.

Another way of relating CIs to hypothesis-testing is as follows: A hypothesis test tells us whether the observed data are consistent with the null hypothesis. A CI tells us which hypotheses are consistent with the data. Another way of putting it is that the p-value gives you a yes or no answer: are the data highly likely (meaning p > 0.05) to have been observed by chance? (Or, alternatively, are we highly likely to mistakenly reject the null hypothesis by chance?) Yes or No. The CIs give you more information: they provide actual effect size (which p-values do not) and they provide an estimate of precision (which p-values do not: how likely are the observed means to differ if we are to repeat the study?). Since the information provided by a p-value of 0.05 is the same as what is provided by a CI of 95%, there is no need to provide p-values when CIs are used (although researchers routinely do so, perhaps because they think that readers cannot interpret CIs). Or, put another way, CIs provide all the information one finds in p-values, *and more*. Hence, the relevance of the proposal, somewhat serious, that p-values should be abolished altogether in favor of CIs (Lang *et al.*, 1998).

Clinical example: the antidepressants and suicide controversy

A humbling example of the misuse of hypothesis-testing statistics, and underuse of effect estimation methods, involves the controversy about whether antidepressants cause suicide. Immediately, two opposite views hardened: opponents of psychiatry saw antidepressants as dangerous killers, and the psychiatric profession circled the wagons, unwilling to admit any validity to the claim of a link to suicidality. An example of the former extreme was the emphasis on specific cases where antidepressant use appeared to be followed by agitation, worsened depression, and suicide. Such cases cannot be dismissed, but they are the weakest kind of evidence. An example of the other extreme was the report, put up with fanfare, by a task force of the American College of Neuropsychopharmacology (ACNP) (American College of Neuropsychopharmacology, 2004) (Table 9.2).

By pooling different studies with each serotonin reuptake inhibitor (SRI) separately, and showing that each of those agents did not reach statistical significance in showing a link with suicide attempts, the ACNP task force claimed that there was *no evidence at all* of such a link. It is difficult to believe that at least some of the distinguished researchers on the task force were unaware of the concept of statistical power, and ignorant of the axiom that failure to disprove the null hypothesis is not proof of it (as discussed in Chapter 7). Nor is it likely that they were unaware of the weakness of a "vote-counting" approach to reviewing the literature (see Chapter 13).

When the same data were analyzed more appropriately, by meta-analysis, the US Food and Drug Administration (FDA) was able to demonstrate not only statistical significance, but a concerning effect size of about twofold increased risk of suicidality (suicide attempts or increased suicidal ideation) with SRIs over placebo (RR = 1.95, 95% CIs 1.28, 2.98). This concerning relative risk needs to be understood in the context of the absolute risk, however, which is where the concept of an NNH becomes useful. The absolute difference between placebo and SRIs was 0.1%. This is a real risk, but obviously a small one absolutely: which is seen when converted to NNH (1/0.01) = 100. Thus, of every one hundred patients treated with antidepressants, one patient would make a suicide attempt attributable to them. One could then compare this risk, with presumed benefit, as I do below.

This is the proper way to analyze such data, not by relying on anecdote to claim massive harm, nor by misusing hypothesis-testing statistics to claim no harm at all. Descriptive statistics tell the true story: there is harm, but it is small. Then the art of medicine takes over: Osler's art of balancing probabilities. The benefits of antidepressants would then need to be weighed against this small, but real, risk.

The TADS study

Another approach was to conduct a larger randomized clinical trial (RCT) to try to answer the question, with a specific plan to look at suicidality as a secondary outcome (unlike all the studies in the FDA database). This led to the National Institute of Mental Health (NIMH)-sponsored Treatment of Adolescent Depression Study (TADS) (March *et al.*, 2004). Even there, though, where no pharmaceutical influence existed based on funding, the investigators appear to underreport the suicidal risks of fluoxetine by overreliance on hypothesis-testing methods.

In that study 479 adolescents were double-blind randomized in a factorial design to fluoxetine vs. cognitive behavioral therapy (CBT) vs. both vs. neither. Response rates were 61% vs. 43% vs. 71% vs. 35%, respectively, with differences being statistically significant. Clinically significant suicidality was present in 29% of children at baseline (more than most previous studies, which is good because it provides a larger number of outcomes for assessment), and worsening suicidal ideation or a suicide attempt was defined as the secondary outcome of "suicide-related adverse events." (No completed suicides occurred in 12 weeks of treatment.) Seven suicide attempts were made, six on fluoxetine. In the abstract, the investigators reported improvement in suicidality in all four groups, without commenting on the differential worsening in the fluoxetine group. The text reported 5.0% (24) suicide-related adverse events, but it did not report the results with RR and CIs. When I analyzed those data that way, one sees the following risk of worsened suicidality: with fluoxetine, RR 1.77 [0.76, 4.15]; with CBT RR 0.85 [0.37, 1.94]. The paper speculates about possible protective benefits with CBT for suicidality, even though the CIs are too wide to infer much probability of such benefit. In contrast, the apparent increase in suicidal risk with fluoxetine, which appears more probable based on the CIs than in the CBT effect, is not discussed in as much detail. The low suicide attempt rate (1.6%, n = 7) is reported, but the overwhelming prevalence with fluoxetine use is not. Using effect estimate methods, the risk of suicide attempts with fluoxetine is RR 6.19

[0.75, 51.0]. Due to the low frequency, this risk is not statistically significant. But hypothesis-testing methods are inappropriate here; use of effect estimation shows a large sixfold risk, which is probably present, and which could be as high as 51-fold.

Hypothesis-testing methods, biased toward the null hypothesis, tells one story; effect estimation methods, less biased and more neutral, tell another. For side effects in general, especially for infrequent ones such as suicidality, the effect estimation stories are closer to reality.

An Oslerian approach to antidepressants and suicide

Recalling Osler's dictum that the art of medicine is the art of balancing probabilities, we can conclude that the antidepressant/suicide controversy is not a question of yes or no, but rather of whether there is a risk, quantifying that risk, and then weighing that risk against benefits.

This effort has not been made systematically, but one researcher made a start in a letter to the editor commenting on the TADS study (Carroll, 2004), noting that the NNH for suicide-related adverse events in the TADS study was 34 (6.9% with fluoxetine versus 4.0% without it). The NNH for suicide attempts was 43 (2.8% with fluoxetine versus 0.45% without it). In contrast, the benefit seen with improvement of depression was more notable; the NNT for fluoxetine was 3.7.

So about four patients need to be treated to improve depression in one of them, while a suicide attempt due to fluoxetine will only occur after 43 patients are treated. This would seem to favor the drug, but we are really comparing apples and oranges: improving depression is fine, but how many deaths due to suicide from the drug are we willing to accept?

One has to now bring in other probabilities besides the actual data from the study (an approach related to Bayesian statistics, see Chapter 14): epidemiological studies indicate that about 8% of suicide attempts end in death. Thus, with an NNH of suicide attempts of 43, the NNH for completed suicide would be 538 (43 divided by 0.08). This would seem to be a very small risk; but it is a serious outcome. Can we balance it by an estimate of prevention of suicide?

The most conservative estimate of lifetime suicide in unipolar major depressive disorder is 2.2%. If we presume that a part of this lifetime rate will occur in adolescence (perhaps 30%), then an adolescent suicide rate of 0.66% might be viable. This produces an NNT for prevention of suicide with fluoxetine, based on the TADS data, of 561 (3.7 divided by 0.0066).

We could also do the same kind of analysis using the FDA database cited previously, which found an NNH for suicide attempts of 100 (higher than the TADS study) (Hammad et al., 2006). If 8% of those patients complete suicide, then the NNH for completed suicide is 1250 (100 divided by 0.08).

So we save one life out of every 561 that we treat, and we take one life out of every 538, or possibly every 1250 patients. Applying Osler's dictum about the art of medicine meaning balancing probabilities, it comes out as a wash, at worst. It is also possible that the actual suicide rates used above are too conservative, and that antidepressants might have somewhat more preventive benefit than suggested above, but even with more benefit, their relative benefit would still be in the NNT range of over 100, which is generally considered minimal.

Overall, then antidepressants have minimal benefits, and minimal risks, it would appear, in relation to suicide.

Lessons learned

At some level, the controversy about antidepressants and suicide had to do with mistaken abuse of hypothesis-testing statistics. The proponents of the association argued that anecdotes were real, and not refuted by the RCTs. They were correct. Their opponents claimed that the amount of risk shown in RCTs was small. They were correct. Both sides erred when they claimed their view was absolutely correct: based on anecdote, one side wanted to view antidepressants as dangerous in general; based on statistical non-significance, the other side wanted to argue there was no effect at all.

Both groups had no adequate comprehension of science, medical statistics, or evidence-based medicine. When effect estimation methods are applied, we see that there is no scientific basis for any controversy. There is a real risk of suicide with antidepressants, but that risk is small, and equal to or less than the probable benefit of prevention of suicide with such agents.

Overall, antidepressants neither cause more death nor do they save lives. If we choose to use them or not, our decisions would then need to be on other grounds (e.g., quality of life, side effects, medical risks). But the suicide question does not push us one way or the other.

Cohort studies

The standard use of effect estimation statistics is in prospective cohort studies. In this case the exposure occurs before the outcome. The main advantages of the prospective cohort study are that researchers do not bias their observations since they state their hypotheses beforehand, before the outcomes have occurred; also researchers usually collect the outcomes systematically in such studies. Thus, although the data are still observational and not randomized, the regression analysis that later follows can use a rich dataset, in which many of the relevant confounding variables are fully and accurately collected.

Classic examples of prospective cohort studies in medicine are the Framingham Heart Study and the Nurses Health Study, both ongoing now for decades, and rich sources of useful knowledge about cardiovascular disease. An example of a psychiatric cohort study, conducted for 5 years, was the recent Systematic Treatment Enhancement Program for Bipolar Disorder (STEP-BD) project.

Chart reviews: pros and cons

Prospective cohort studies are expensive and time-consuming. The 5-year STEP-BD project cost about $20 million. There are many, many more important medical questions that need to be answered than can be approached either by RCTs or prospective cohort studies. Hence we are forced to rely, in some questions, at some phases of the scientific research process, on retrospective cohort studies. Here the outcomes have already occurred, and thus there is more liability to bias on the part of researchers looking for the causes that may have led to those outcomes.

A classic example of a retrospective cohort study is the case-control paradigm. In this kind of study, cases with an outcome (e.g., lung cancer) are compared with controls who do not have the outcome (no lung cancer). The two groups are then compared on an exposure (e.g., rates of cigarette smoking). The important issue is to try to match the case and control groups as much as possible on all possible factors except for the experimental variable of interest. This is usually technically infeasible beyond a few basic features such as age, gender, ethnicity, and similar variables. The risks of confounding bias are very high. Regression analysis can help reduce confounding bias in a large enough sample, but one is often faced with a lack of adequate data previously collected on many relevant confounding variables.

All these limitations given, it is still relevant that retrospective cohort studies are important sources of scientific evidence and that they are often correct. For instance, the relationship between cigarette smoking and lung cancer was almost completely established in the 1950s and 1960s based on retrospective case-control studies, even without any statistical regression analysis (which had not yet been developed).

Despite a long period of criticism of those data by skeptics, those case-control results have stood up to the test of other better designed studies and analyses.

Nonetheless, the limitations of retrospective cohort study deserve some examination.

Limitations of retrospective observational studies

One of these limitations, especially relevant for psychiatric research, is *recall bias*, the fact that people have poor memories for their medical history. In one study, patients were asked to recall their past treatments with antidepressants for up to five years; these recollections were then compared to the actual documented treatments kept by the same investigators in their patient charts. The researchers found that patients recalled 80% of treatments received in the prior year, which may not seem bad; but by 5 years, they only recalled 67% of treatments received (Posternak and Zimmerman, 2003). Since some chart reviews extend back decades, we can expect that we are only getting about half the story if we rely mainly on patient's self-report. While this is a problem, there is also a reality: prospective studies lasting decades in duration will not be available for most of the medical questions that we need to answer. So again, using *real* (not ivory-tower) evidence-based medicine (EBM): *some data, any data, properly analyzed, are better than no data*. I would view this glass as half full, and take the information available in chart reviews, with the appropriate level of caution; I would not, as many academics do, see it as half empty and thus reject such studies as worthless.

Another example of recall bias relates to diagnosis. A major depressive episode is usually painful and patients know they are sick: they do not lack insight into depression. Thus, one would expect reasonably good recall of having experienced severe depression in the past. In a study, however, researchers interviewed 45 patients who had been hospitalized 25 years earlier for a major depressive episode (Andrews *et al.*, 1999). Twenty-five years later, 70% recalled being depressed and only 52% were able to give sufficient detail for researchers to be able to fully identify sufficient criteria to meet the severity of a full major depressive episode. So, even with hospitalized depression, 30% of patients do not recall the symptoms at all decades later, and only about 50% recall the episode in detail.

The HRT study

The best recent example of the risks of observational research is the experience of the medical community with estrogenic hormone replacement therapy (HRT) in postmenopausal women. All evidence short of RCTs – multiple large prospective cohort studies, many retrospective cohort studies, and the individual clinical experience of the majority of physicians and specialists – agreed that HRT was beneficial in many ways (for osteoporosis, mood, memory) and not harmful. A large RCT by the Women's Health Initiative (WHI) investigators disproved this belief: the treatment was not effective in any demonstrable way, and it caused harm by increasing the risk of certain cancers. The WHI study also was an observational prospective cohort study, and thus it provided the unique opportunity to compare the best non-randomized (prospective cohort) and randomized data of the same topic in the same sample. This comparison showed that observational data (even under the best conditions) inflates efficacy compared to RCTs (Prentice *et al.*, 2006).

Many clinicians are still disturbed by the results of the Women's Health Initiative RCT; some insist that certain subgroups had benefit, which may be the case, although this possibility needs to be interpreted with the caution that is due subgroup analysis (see Chapter 8). But, in the end, this experience is an important cautionary tale about the deep and profound reality of confounding bias, and the limitations of our ability to observe what is really the case in our daily clinical experience.

The benefits of observational research

The case against observational studies should not be overstated, however. Ivory-tower EBM proponents tend to assume that observational studies systematically overestimate effect sizes compared to RCTs in many different conditions and settings. In fact, this kind of generic overestimation has not been empirically shown. One review that assessed the matter came to the opposite conclusion (Benson and Hartz, 2000). That analysis looked at 136 studies of 19 treatments in a range of medical specialties (from cardiology to psychiatry); it found that only 2 of the 19 analyses showed inflated effect sizes with observational studies compared to RCTs. In most cases, in fact, RCTs only confirmed what observational studies had already found. Perhaps this consistency may relate more to high-quality observational studies (prospective cohort studies) than other observational data, but it should be a source of caution for those who would throw away all knowledge except those studies anointed with placebos.

Randomized clinical trials are the gold standard, and the most valid kind of knowledge. But they have their limits. Where they cannot be conducted, observational research, properly understood, is a linchpin of medical knowledge.

10

Causation

What does causation mean?

The whole point of all of the foregoing – of all of the ins and outs of randomized clinical trials (RCTs), and the rigors of regression – is to produce results that allow us to say that something causes something else. All of statistics until this point is about allowing us to infer causation, to make us feel ready to do so. But those efforts – RCTs and regression and the like – do not automatically allow us to infer causation. Causation itself is a separate matter, one which we need to consider, a third hurdle (after bias and chance) which we must pass before we can say we are finished.

Hume's fallacy

Causation is essentially a philosophical, not a statistical, problem. Here we see again a key spot where statistics itself does not provide the answers, but we must go outside statistics in order to understand statistics.

The concept of causation may seem simple initially. My daughter, looking over my shoulder at this chapter title, read: "What does causation mean? Well, it means that something caused something. Right?" "Well, yes," I replied. "That's simple, then," she said. "Even an 8-year-old can figure that out."

It seems simple. If I throw a brick at a window, the window breaks: the brick *caused* the window to break. The sun rises every morning and night is replaced by day. The sun *causes* daylight. The word comes from the Latin *causa*, which throws little light on its meaning, except perhaps that it also means "reason." A cause is a reason, but, as we also know by common sense, there are many reasons for many things. There is not just one reason in every case that causes something to happen. The first common sense intuition we must then recognize is that causation can mean *a* cause and it can mean *many* causes. It does not necessarily mean *the* cause (Doll, 2002).

The instincts of common sense were long ago dethroned in the eighteenth century by the philosopher David Hume, who noted that our intuitions about one thing causing another involved an empirical "constant conjunction" of the two events, but no inherent metaphysical link between the two. Every day, the sun rises. A day passes, the sun rises again. There is a constant conjunction; but this in no way proves that some day the sun might not rise: we can call this *Hume's fallacy*.

In other words, observations in the real world cannot prove that one thing causes another; *induction* fails. Hume's critique led many philosophers to search for *deduction* of causality, as in mathematical proofs. Yet the force of his arguments for activities in the world of time and space, such as science, has not lessened, and they are central to understanding the uses and limits of statistics in medicine and psychiatry. (I will give more attention to this matter in the next Chapter 11.)

The tobacco wars

These two facts – the recognition that induction can be faulty, and the mistaken assumption that causation has to imply *the* cause – have led to much unnecessary scientific conflict over the years. Even Ronald Fisher, the brilliant founder of modern statistics, did not fathom it. In his later life (the 1950s and 1960s), Fisher became a loud critic of those who used his methods to suggest a link between cigarette smoking and lung cancer. Of course, there is no one-to-one connection. Many smokers never develop lung cancer, and some people develop lung cancer who never smoke. These facts led Fisher to doubt the claimed association. Cigarette smoking did not *cause* lung cancer, Fisher argued; because he thought that had to be *the* cause, the one and only cause, with no other causes. As noted previously (Chapter 7), part of Fisher's scientific concern also was that he felt that the concept of *statistical significance* (p-values) could only be applied in the setting of an RCT. Its application in a completely observational setting, as with cigarette smoking, seemed to him inappropriate. Fisher's view was partly limited by the fact that he did not appreciate the rise of a new discipline, related to but different from statistics: the field of clinical epidemiology. Its founder, A. Bradford Hill, was on the other side of this debate of giants. The conflict over cigarette smoking led Hill to formulate a list of factors that help us in understanding causation.

We can now, with the advantage of hindsight, look back on this debate and use it to inform how we understand current debates. Today almost everyone accepts that cigarette smoking causes lung cancer; it is not the *only* cause (other environmental toxins can do so too, and in rare cases purely genetic causation occurs), but it is the *main* cause. In 1950, the first strong piece of evidence to support the link was a case-control study conducted in London. In that study, Hill and his colleague Richard Doll examined 20 London hospitals and identified 709 patients with lung cancer, and matched them by age and gender to 709 patients without lung cancer. They found an association between how many cigarettes had been reported to be smoked and lung cancer. It was not definitive, it was not a 100% connection, but it was present far beyond what might be expected by chance. The key issue was bias. The term "confounding bias" had not been invented yet, but the concept was out there: could there be other causes of the apparent relationship?

Statistics versus epidemiology

Hill and Doll argued that other causes that could completely, or almost completely, explain their findings were implausible. But they had many weaknesses in their claim. First, no animal studies had identified specific carcinogens in cigarette smoke. Second, argued the tobacco industry, their main source of data was patient recall about past smoking habits: patient recall is obviously known to be faulty. Third, again said the industry, other plausible causes existed, such as environmental pollution, which had increased in the same time frame, and which correlated with the finding that lung cancer was present more in cities than in rural areas. Fisher finally weighed in by adding the other possibility of genetic susceptibility, which he had identified as present in twin studies.

Hill and Doll faced a problem: how can you prove causation in clinical epidemiology? Put another way, how can you prove that anything causes anything else when you are dealing with human beings? With animals, one could control for genetics by breeding for specific genetic types; one can control the environment in a laboratory as well so that animals can be studied such that they only differ on one feature (the experimental question). But such experiments are not feasible nor ethical with humans. How can we ever prove that something causes a disease in humans?

This is the problem of clinical epidemiology. And the conflict between Fisher and Hill shows that statistics are not enough. The numbers can never give the complete answer, *because they are never definitive*. Statistics, by nature, are never absolute: they are about measuring the probability of error; they can never remove error.

Thus, if one wants to be certain, or very very certain, as in the case where human liberties are being restricted (your rights to cigarette smoking are curtailed, for instance), we seem to have a problem. Fisher, seeing the statistical limits of certainty, felt that it would be hard to prove causation in medical disease. Hill, knowing those same limits, set out to devise a solution.

We have here also, by the way, the source of the philosophical conflict between the two fields of statistics and clinical epidemiology. This is often not obvious to doctors or clinicians, but it is relevant to them. For, with many research questions, if clinicians ask a statistician they will get a different answer than if they ask an epidemiologist; this can especially be the case when one is concerned with interpreting a number of different studies, as in the Fisher versus Hill debate. One solution is to recognize a division of labor: statisticians are best trained in analyzing the results of a study and in focusing on the risks of chance; epidemiologists are best trained in designing studies and in focusing on the risks of bias. Or put another way, statisticians are most trained in the conduct of RCTs and tend to think with hypothesis-testing methods; epidemiologists are most trained in the conduct of observational cohort studies and tend to think with descriptive effect estimation methods. The two groups are the Red Sox and Yankees of medical research, and clinicians need to be willing to speak with and understand the perspectives of both of them.

Hill's concepts of causation

Now let's turn to what Hill had to say about causation, beginning with a few words about the man. A. Bradford Hill is generally seen as the founder of modern medical epidemiology; modern medicine would be inconceivable without him, and so too with medical statistics. If Fisher invented the ideas, such as randomization, Hill applied them to clinical medicine, and worked out their meaning in that context. A single achievement of his would have sufficed to mark the successful career of another man, but Hill was truly revolutionary in his impact. He brought randomization to clinical medical research, conducting the first RCT in 1948 on streptomycin for pneumonia. This, in itself, is like the French Revolution for modern medicine. Yet, in addition to showing how RCTs can bring us closer to the truth – in a way, founding medical statistics in the process – he also realized that much of medicine was not amenable to RCTs, and thus, he showed us how to apply statistical methods effectively in observational settings – thus founding clinical epidemiology in the process. This would be the second great revolution of modern medicine. And, in the process, by demonstrating the link between cigarette smoking and lung cancer, Hill rooted out the most deadly preventable illness of the modern era.

With that background, we can listen to what he had to say about the evidence needed to conclude that causation is present in clinical research.

It is a commonplace in statistics that association does not necessarily imply causation. The question then is: when does it? This was the topic of a presidential address Hill gave to the Royal Society of Medicine in London: "The environment and disease: association or causation?" (Hill, 1965). Hill first abjures "a philosophical discussion of the meaning of 'causation,'" which we leave for the next chapter. He then defines the practical question for physicians as "whether the frequency of the undesirable event B will be influenced by a change in the environmental feature A." If we observe an association through observation, unlikely to have occurred by chance, the question is how we can then claim causation. Hill then enumerates the ingredients of causation:

1. *Strength of the association.* Smoking increases the likelihood of lung cancer about tenfold, while it increases the likelihood of heart attack about twofold. A very large effect, such as tenfold or higher, should be seen as strong evidence of causation, Hill argues, unless one can identify some other feature (a confounding factor) directly associated with the proposed cause. With such a large effect size, confounding factors should be relatively easy to detect, says Hill, thus allowing us "to reject the vague contention of the armchair critic 'you can't prove it, there *may* be such a feature.'" (Surely he was thinking of Ronald Fisher here.)

   The reverse does not hold: "We must not be too ready to dismiss a cause-and-effect hypothesis merely on the grounds that the observed association appears to be slight. There are many occasions in medicine when this is in truth so. Relatively few persons harbouring the meningococcus fall sick of meningococcal meningitis." A strong association makes causation likely; a weak association does not, by itself, make causation unlikely.

2. *Consistency of the association.* This reflects replication – "Has it been repeatedly observed by different persons, in different places, circumstances and times?" The key to replication, though, is not to replicate using *the exact same* methods, but rather to replicate using *different* methods. For instance, biased studies are easily replicated; bias reflects *systematic* error, so repetition of a biased study will *systematically* produce the same error. Thus, one non-randomized observational study found that antidepressant discontinuation in bipolar depression led to depressive recurrence (Altshuler *et al.*, 2003). Another non-randomized observational study "replicated" the same finding (Joffe *et al.*, 2005). The researchers mistakenly viewed this as strengthening inference of causation. What would strengthen the observational finding would be if randomized data found the same result (which did not occur [Ghaemi *et al.*, 2008b]). In the case of RCTs, replication by other RCTs would count as improving strength of causation, but again preferably with some differences, such as different dosages or somewhat different patient populations.

   Again, since no feature is an essential feature of causation, replication is not a *sine qua non*: "there will be occasions when repetition is absent or impossible and yet we should not hesitate to draw conclusions." This occurs with rare events: if lamotrigine causes Stevens-Johnson syndrome in about 1 in 1000 persons, statistically significant replication would require a study in which the drug is given to about 3200 persons, assuming a small standard deviation. This kind of replication is not only unethical, but impossible, another example of the limitations of the p-value approach to statistics, another reason to realize that the concept of "statistical significance" is very limited in its meaning. Causation is a much more important, and inclusive, concept.

3. *Specificity of the association.* Smoking causes lung cancer, not hives. However, this factor should not be overemphasized because some exposures can cause many effects: smoking turns out to increase the risk of a range of cancers, not just limited to the lungs. Again, a positive finding rules in causation much more strongly than a negative finding would rule

it out: "if specificity exists we may be able to draw conclusions without hesitation; if it is not apparent, we are not thereby necessarily left sitting irresolutely on the fence."

4. *Temporality.* In the world of time and space, causes precede effects, so unidirectionality in time is important. Fisher once argued that the association between lung cancer and smoking could conceivably be causative in either direction: perhaps persons with lung cancer were more inclined to smoke, so as to reduce pulmonary irritation caused by their cancers. Yet, Hill could show that most smokers began their habit in their youth, long before they developed lung cancer.

5. *Biological gradient.* This is the dose–response relationship – the more one smokes, the higher the rate of lung cancer. The presence of such a gradient allows one to identify a clear and often linear causative relationship. More complex non-linear relationships can exist, however, such that again, this factor is not definitive, and its absence does not rule out causation.

6. *Plausibility.* It is helpful, writes Hill, if the causative inference is biologically plausible. This is a weak criterion, since "what is biologically plausible depends on the biological knowledge of the day," which in turn often depends on the presence or absence of clinical/observational suggestions of topics for biological research. There is a vicious circle here: before Hill's work, since no one had raised seriously the association between cigarette smoking and lung cancer, biological researchers would not have been exposed to the idea that it should be studied. Thus, when Hill and his group identified the clinical association, they were faced with a biological abyss of nothingness – no biological research was available to explain their findings. Indeed, it took decades to come. Here is where Hill makes an important claim, which dates back to Hippocrates, and which conflicts with many of the assumptions of biological researchers: clinical observation trumps biology, not vice versa. We should believe our clinical eyes, sharpened by the lenses of statistics and epidemiology; we should not reject what we see just because our biological theories do not yet explain them. Hill quotes the physician Arthur Conan Doyle's wise medical advice, put in the mouth of Sherlock Holmes: "When you have eliminated the impossible, whatever remains, *however improbable*, must be the truth."

7. *Coherence.* While one must be open to observations that await confirmation by biological research as above, we should also put our observations in the context of what is reasonably well proven biologically: "the cause-and-effect interpretation of our data should not seriously conflict with the generally known facts of the natural history and biology of the disease." One would not want to invoke an extraterrestrial cause of medical disease, for instance. This is not altogether irrelevant: in recent years, a generally sane full professor of psychiatry at Harvard observed cases of persons with sexual trauma who attributed those events to alien abduction. After collecting a number of cases, the psychiatrist argued (in a best-selling book) for a cause-and-effect relationship on standard scientific grounds (Mack, 1995). Applying Hill's advice, there was an association; the effect size was there; it was consistent, apparently specific, obeyed temporality of cause and effect, and even appeared to have a dose-and-effect relationship (people who reported longer periods of abduction experienced more post-traumatic stress symptoms). But it was radically incoherent with the minimal facts of human biology.

Thus coherence is not a minor matter, though it might seem somewhat trivial. If a proposed cause-and-effect relationship is illogical, it is a weak proposal; and many logical relationships are incoherent metaphysically.

8. *Experiment.* This is the whole of scientific causation outside of the world of human beings, i.e., outside of clinical research. In basic research, with cells or animals or ions, one can conduct a true experiment. By holding all aspects of the environment stable except for one factor, one can definitively conclude that X causes Y. With humans, this kind of environmental control is unethical and infeasible. In effect, RCTs are experiments with humans. They are how we can get at this aspect of causation, though again only with probability (though often quite high), not absolute certainty (unlike, perhaps, completely controlled animal experiments). Because he was speaking to epidemiologists rather than statisticians, Hill did not emphasize the role of RCTs as experiment in his address. He rather pointed out that sometimes we can make interventions that can help support causation: for instance, did the removal of an exposure prevent further cases of disease? This would support a causative relationship.

Perhaps Hill also downplayed the role of RCTs in experimentation because of his debate with Fisher. Fisher was saying that RCTs were a *sine qua non* of causation; Hill wanted to argue otherwise, partly because RCTs were unethical or infeasible for many important topics, such as cigarette smoking.

As a more general conceptual matter, I would tend to agree with Fisher, and I think we should be more definitive than Hill: I would not place experiment eighth on the list of causation; I would define it as meaning RCTs, *where feasible* (thus in agreement with Hill in regards to cigarette smoking), and I would place it first, because it gives us the strongest evidence (though again it is not definitive).

Recall that even here no criterion is essential. The absence of RCTs does not rule out causation, and their presence is not required to infer causation. Again, since this reflects human experimentation, questions of feasibility and ethics arise: no RCT ever demonstrated that cigarette smoking causes lung cancer, nor can or should it. We would have to randomize two large groups of people, probably at least 5000 in each arm, to smoke or not smoke for about 10–20 years, and then assess incurable lung cancer as the outcome. Enough said.

9. *Analogy.* This feature of causation deserves to be last, since like coherence, though it is relevant, it can be trivial. Hill notes that since rubella, for instance, is associated with pregnancy-related malformations, some other viruses can be expected to pose similar risks.

These are Hill's nine features of causation, given in the order of importance which he used. I would reorder them as in Table 10.1.

Often called the "Hill criteria," we should keep in mind that causation is not a matter of checklists and criteria. It is rather a conceptual problem, as Hume demonstrated. And, one needs to weigh different features of the evidence, clinical and biological, in coming to conclusions regarding causation. Even with all this effort, as Hume pointed out long ago, causation is still usually a matter of a high level of probability, rather than absolute certainty (see Chapter 11).

Sir Richard Doll, Hill's younger associate, has suggested reducing this list to four key features, which if met on a specific topic, should be definitive proof of causation: "With the experience that we now have of thousands of epidemiological studies, we can conclude that large relative risks – on the order of $> 20:1$ – with evidence of a dose-response relationship, that cannot be explained by methodological bias or reasonably be attributed to chance (with p-levels of $< 1 \times 10^{-6}$) are in themselves adequate proof of a causal relationship." (Doll,

Table 10.1. A. Bradford Hill's features of causation

1. Experiment (RCTs)
2. Strength of an association (Effect size)
3. Consistency of an association (Replication)
4. Specificity
5. Relationship in time (Cause precedes effect)
6. Biological gradient (Dose–response relationship)
7. Biological plausibility
8. Coherence of the evidence
9. Reasoning by analogy

RCTs = randomized clinical trials.
From A. B. Hill, *Principles of Medical Statistics*, 9th edn, 1971. With permission from Oxford University Press.

2002; p. 512.) Here are the four factors, then: (a) a huge relative risk; (b) a dose–response relationship; (c) minimal bias; and (d) tiny likelihood by chance (p < 0.00001). Doll points out that the 1950 cigarette smoking data met these criteria; this is sobering, since a half century more had to pass before the force of this truth could overcome the power of organized lies produced by the tobacco industry (proving the importance of the politics of research; see Chapter 17). It is also sobering, however, because Doll is arguing for agreement on a high threshold. Today, as he admits, most of our evidence falls far below this threshold; hence the need for attention to the other features identified by Hill. Thus, a small relative risk of cancer caused by estrogenic contraceptives can still be convincing, when supplemented by animal studies demonstrating similar effects.

Biological causation

We might contrast Hill's features of causation – which is the core of epidemiology and a conceptual linchpin for the evidence-based medicine (EBM) approach – with the traditional biological approach in medicine encapsulated in Koch's postulates for causation. In the beginning of the bacterial era, the nineteenth-century German physician Robert Koch argued that we could conclude that a bacterial agent caused a particular disease if the following postulates are met:

1. "Whenever an agent was cultured, the disease was there.

2. Whenever the disease was not there, the agent could not be cultured.

3. When the agent was removed, the disease went away." (Salsburg, 2001; p. 186.)

As Salsburg points out, this definition of causation is similar to what the philosopher Bertrand Russell would later call "material implication" (see Chapter 11). It can apply to some (not all) infectious diseases in which the bacterial agent is *necessary and sufficient* to cause disease. But many causes are necessary but not sufficient; others are sufficient but not necessary. Some causes are neither necessary nor sufficient, but they are still causes. Cigarette smoking is in this last category: one can get lung cancer without smoking; one can smoke without getting lung cancer. But it is a cause. The biological definition of causation fails for most chronic medical illnesses that have more than one cause. This was the problem Hill was trying to solve.

Causation is a concept, not a number

Hill ended his discussion by reminding us that causation is not about chance and the use of statistics: it is a conceptual matter. Again, p-values and statistical significance are not relevant. This common misconception is such a major problem in medical statistics, in my view, that I wish to let Hill (1965) speak for himself on this matter, beckoning from 1965 to new generations of clinicians and researchers:

> Between the two world wars there was a strong case for emphasizing to the clinician and other research workers the importance of not overlooking the play of chance upon their data. Perhaps too often generalities were based upon two men and a laboratory dog while the treatment of choice was deduced from a difference between two bedfuls of patients and might easily have no true meaning. It was therefore a useful corrective for statisticians to stress, and to teach the need for, tests of significance merely to serve as guides to caution before drawing a conclusion, before inflating the particular to the general.
>
> I wonder whether the pendulum has not swung too far – not only with the attentive pupils but even with the statisticians themselves. To decline to draw conclusions without standard errors can surely be just as silly? ... there are innumerable situations in which [tests of significance] are totally unnecessary – because the difference is grotesquely obvious, because it is negligible, or because, whether it be formally significant or not, it is too small to be of any practical importance. What is worse the glitter of the t table diverts attention from the inadequacies of the fare ...
>
> Of course I exaggerate. Yet too often I suspect we waste a great deal of time, we grasp the shadow and lose the substance, we weaken our capacity to interpret data and to take reasonable decisions whatever the value of P. And far too often we deduce 'no difference' from 'no significant difference.' Like fire, the χ^2 test is an excellent servant and a bad master.

Practical causation

A final point is in order, one on which Hill ends his address: causation is not a theoretical matter for medicine; it is a practical one. The reason I infer, or do not infer, causation is because I will, or will not, give drug X to patient Y. The threshold for inferring causation may differ depending on the practical matter at hand. If I am thinking of giving a drug with major toxicities, I will want many, if not most, of Hill's features to be met. If I am the Surgeon General, and I am thinking of restricting the civil rights of citizens to smoke in restaurants, I will want many, if not most, of Hill's features to be met. However, if I am a researcher inferring causation on a matter of little practical importance (e.g., that sunlight exposure decreases latency to REM sleep), a lower threshold for acceptance of causation will not harm anyone. The truth will remain the truth, wherever we put our thresholds for causation, but we should not immobilize ourselves when important practical questions need to be answered (Bayesian statistics provides a way to manage this problem; see Chapter 14). We still need to decide, one way or the other, and *not* deciding, as the philosopher William James reminded us so well, is one way of deciding (the easy, passive way) (James, 1956 [1897]). Recall that statistics is not meant to keep us from inferring causation, or doing something, because we are not absolutely, or near absolutely certain. Statistics is merely a way, as Laplace put it, of quantifying, rather than ignoring, error. How much error we are willing to accept depends on the circumstances. Here is Hill (1965):

…on relatively slight evidence we might decide to restrict the use of a drug for early-morning sickness in pregnant women. If we are wrong in deducing causation from association no great harm will be done. The good lady and the pharmaceutical industry will doubtless survive. … All scientific work is incomplete – whether it be observational or experimental. All scientific work is liable to be upset or modified by advancing knowledge. That does not confer upon us a freedom to ignore the knowledge we already have, or to postpone the action that it appears to demand at a given time.

Who knows, asked Robert Browning, but the world may end tonight? True, but on available evidence most of us make ready to commute on the 8.30 next day.

Replication and the wish to believe

To this point, readers will be aware that if statistics are well understood, both conceptually and historically, no single report can be seen as definitive. Replication is a key feature for attributing causation to any medical claim. If nothing else, the cigarette smoking and lung cancer controversy between Fisher and Hill should have taught us this fact. History is poorly studied, however, and statistics are little understood conceptually.

As a result, it seems to be the case that first impressions, from initial studies or early reports, have staying power in the consciousness of clinicians.

This phenomenon has begun to be documented empirically. In one analysis (Ioannidis, 2005), researchers examined 49 highly cited original clinical research studies, most of which claimed benefit with a treatment. Later studies contradicted the initial findings in 16%, or found a smaller effect size of benefit in another 16%. Forty-four percent were replicated, and 24% were never re-examined. Initial reports were more likely to be later contradicted if they were non-randomized (5/6, 83%, of non-randomized studies were contradicted versus only 9/39, 23%, of RCTs), or if they were randomized but small in sample size.

If we apply Hill's feature of replication, over half of highly cited clinical research studies fail the test. This would be enough to give us pause if it were not the case that it seems that clinicians and researchers appear more readily to accept positive than negative replication. Clinical opinions persist, even after they have been studied and refuted (Tatsioni *et al.*, 2007). Those investigators examined the view that vitamin E supplementation has cardiovascular benefits, a perspective fostered by reports from large epidemiological studies in 1993. Other non-randomized studies also found benefit, as did one RCT in 2002. But the largest and best designed study found no benefit in 2000, and a meta-analysis of all these studies in 2004 also found no benefit, instead finding increased risk of death at high vitamin E doses. The authors analyzed studies published in the year 1997, so that they were written before most of the RCTs, compared to later articles in 2005 after the publication of clear contradiction of the initial hypothesis of benefit. Although articles written in 1997 were much less unfavorable (2%) to vitamin E than articles written in 2005 (34%), the authors noted that 50% of articles in 2005 continued to favorably cite the earlier literature, by then disproven. They found similar patterns with initial studies of benefit, later disproven, with beta-carotene for cancer and estrogen for dementia.

The researchers noted that specialty, more so than generalist, journals tended to continue to publish favorable articles about the disproven treatments. They also observed:

> In the evaluation of counterarguments, we encountered almost any source of bias, genuine diversity, and biological reasoning invoked to defend the original observations … consistent with a belief that is defended at all cost. The defense of the

observations was persistent, despite the availability of very strong contradicting randomized evidence on the same topic. Thus, one wonders whether any contradicted associations may ever be entirely abandoned ... For most associations and questions of medical interest, either no randomized data exist, or the randomized evidence is minimal and of poor quality.

(Tatsioni *et al.*, 2007)

Though perhaps disappointed, a half century after their debates, I do not think Hill and Fisher would be surprised.

A philosophy of statistics

Every truth ... is an error that has been corrected.

Alexandre Kojeve (Kojeve, 1980; p. 187)

Statistics, as a discipline, does not exist in a vacuum. It is a reflection of our views on science, and thus how it is understood and how it is used depends on what we mean by science. Most statistics texts do not discuss these matters, or if they do, they are perfunctory. But it is important for all involved (statisticians and clinicians) to appreciate their assumptions, and to have some rationale for them.

Cultural positivism

Most doctors and clinicians have an unconscious philosophy of science, imbibed from the larger culture: positivism. Positivism is the view that science is the accumulation of facts. Fact upon fact produces scientific laws. Holding sway through much of the nineteenth and twentieth centuries, the positivistic view of science has seeped into our bones. Beginning in the late nineteenth century, and more definitely after the 1960s, philosophers of science have shown that "facts" do not exist as independent entities; they are tied to theories and hypotheses. Facts cannot be separated from theories; science involves deduction, and not just induction.

The nineteenth-century American philosopher Charles Sanders Peirce, who was a practicing physicist, knew what was involved in the actual practice of science: the scientist has a hypothesis, a theory; this theory might have been based on previous studies, or it might simply be imagined wholecloth (Peirce called this "abduction"); the scientist then tries to verify or refute his theory by facts (either passively through observation or actively through experiment). In this way, no facts are observed without a preceding hypothesis. So facts are "theory-laden"; between fact and theory no sharp line can be drawn (Jaspers, 1997 [1959]).

Verify or refute?

This hypothesis–fact relationship leaves us with a dilemma: in testing our hypotheses, which is more important: verification or refutation? The positivistic view was biased in favor of confirming theories: fact was placed upon fact to verify theories (another name for this view of science is "verificationism"). In the mid twentieth century, Karl Popper rejected positivism by privileging refutation over confirmation: a single negative result was definitive – it refuted a hypothesis – while any positive result was always provisional – it never definitively proves a hypothesis, because it can always be refuted by a negative result. Let us examine Popper's views, and how they apply to different approaches to statistics, more closely.

Karl Popper's philosophy of science

I think it would be fair to argue that in today's world of science and medical research, the assumed philosophy of science (sometimes explicit) is that of the philosopher Karl Popper (Popper, 1959). Popper sought to provide a deductive definition of science to replace the more traditional inductive definition. In the older view, science seemed to involve the accumulation of facts; the more facts, the more science. The problem with this inductive view can be traced back to David Hume, who showed that this approach could never, with complete certainty, prove anything (see Chapter 10). Popper sought complete certainty for science, and he thought he had it with Einstein's discoveries. Einstein was able to make certain predictions based on his theories; if those predictions were wrong, then his theory was wrong. Only one mistake was required to disprove his entire theory. Popper argued that science could best be understood as an activity whose theories could be definitively disproved, but never definitively proven. The best scientific theories, then, would be those which would make falsifiable propositions, and, if not falsified, then those theories might be true. Popper specified Freud and Marx for blame for having claimed to provide scientific theories when in fact their ideas were in no way falsifiable. This approach has become quite popular among modern scientists. Freud and Marx are, in some sense, easy targets; Darwin's theory could just as well be rejected for being unfalsifiable. Ultimately, Popper did not solve the Humean riddle, for Popper's view tells us not which theories are true, but which ones are not.

The limits of refutation

We might summarize that contemporary views of science (heavily influenced by Popper) are focused on hypothesis-testing by refutation. We see this philosophy reflected in statistics, especially in the whole concept of the importance of the p-value and the idea of trying to refute the null hypothesis (see Chapter 7).

My own view is that this refutationism is as wrong as the old verificationism, because no single refutation is definitive. One can have positive results after negative results; what then to make of the original negative results? In statistics, this overemphasis on refutation leads to overuse of p-values, while appropriate appreciation of positive results would lead us to a different kind of statistics (descriptive effect size oriented methods, see Chapter 9).

Charles Peirce's philosophy of science

This leads to an inductive philosophy of science, like that of Charles Peirce (Peirce, 1958), but not exactly in the traditional sense. Peirce accepted induction as the method of science, acknowledged that it led to increasing probabilities of truth, and argued that these probabilities reached the limits of certainty so closely that it was mathematically meaningless to deny certainty to them at a certain point of accumulated evidence. Peirce also added that this accumulation of near-certain inductive knowledge was a process that spanned generations of scientists and that the community of scientists which added to this fund of knowledge would eventually reach consensus on what was likely to be true based on those data.

Causation again

We can now return to that key philosophical aspect of statistics: the problem of causation. In Chapter 10, I reviewed the basic idea of the eighteenth-century philosopher David Hume, arguing that inductive inference did not lead to absolute certainty of causation. The philosopher Bertrand Russell tried to provide another way of looking at the question with his notion of "material implication." Russell argued that if A causes B, we are saying that A "materially implies" B. In other words, there is something in A that is also entailed in B (Salsburg, 2001). He distinguished this material implication from the symbolic nature of other logical relationships (such as conjunction – the "and" relationship – or disjunction – the "or" relationship). When we say, "if A, then B," the "if, then" relationship is not purely symbolic, but has some material basis. This was Russell's view; it does not solve the problem of causation but it suggests a way of thinking about causation that entails that the idea is not a matter of purely symbolic logic, but perhaps an empirical matter.

A final way of thinking about causation – besides Hume's description of induction, and Russell's logical concept of material implication – is a scientific perspective that can be traced to one of the French founders of nineteenth-century experimental medicine, Claude Bernard (Olmsted, 1952). Bernard held that we could conclude that A causes B by conducting an experiment in which all conditions are held constant except A, and showing that B follows. Such proof of causation then is based on being able to control all factors except one, the experimental factor. This is, in practice, difficult to do in biology and medicine, and much more feasible in inorganic sciences such as physics and chemistry. But it can be done. For instance, we have the technology today to conduct animal studies in which the entire animal genome is fixed beforehand; animals can be genetically bred to produce a certain genetic state and they can all be identical in that genetic state; then we can control the animals' environment from birth until death. In that kind of controlled setting, where all genetic and environmental factors are controlled, Bernard's definition of experimental causation may hold.

Such causation is unethical and infeasible with human beings. The closest we get to it is with randomization. As discussed throughout this book, randomization with human beings, though reducing much uncertainty, never reduces all uncertainty, and thus we cannot achieve absolute causation. The importance of randomized clinical trials (RCTs) in getting us very much closer to causation might be highlighted by realizing that they are the closest human approximation to Bernard's *experimental causation*. Fisher was right in emphasizing the need for RCTs in asserting causation, and Hill was right in recognizing the benefits of other features of research, in addition to experimentation with RCTs, so as to reduce uncertainty even further.

The general versus the individual
Another philosophical aspect about statistics is how it reflects the general as opposed to the individual. The Belgian thinker Quetelet recognized the issue in the 1840s; he "knew that individuals' characteristics could not be represented by a deterministic law, but he believed that averages over groups could be so represented." (Stigler, 1986; p. 172.) About half a century later, German philosophers (Wilhelm Windelband and Heinrich Rickert) made this general distinction the basis for their understanding of the nature and limits of science: science consists of general laws; it stops short of the unique and individual. They said there were two kinds of knowledge: nosographic (science – general, statistical, group-based) and idiographic (individual and unique for each particular case). Science "explained" (*Erklaren*) general laws; philosophy and the humanities "understood" (*Verstehen*) the unique characteristics of individuals (Makkreel, 1992).

This criticism of statistics, so often used by modern critics of evidence-based medicine (EBM), was present from the very beginning of the effort (in the mid nineteenth century) to apply statistics to human beings (as in experimental psychology), as opposed to limiting it to mathematics, astronomy, and physics (as had previously been the case). Here is an example from Auguste Comte attacking the statistician Poisson who in 1835 had suggested there might be legal uses for statistics: "The application of this calculus to matters of morality is repugnant to the soul. It amounts, for example, to representing the truth of a verdict by a number, to thus treat men as if they were dice, each with many faces, some for error, some for truth." (Stigler, 1986; p. 194.)

This history reminds me of an exchange I recently had, one that became somewhat heated, during a symposium in the annual convention of the American Psychiatric Association. I and others had reviewed RCTs showing that antidepressants were hardly effective in bipolar depression; one of the discussants, who had previously supported their use, had to bow to the data, but he ended his presentation by declaring forcefully: "Antidepressants may not be as great as we had hoped, but, in the end, your individual experience as a practitioner and that of the patient trumps everything!" Raucous applause followed from the packed audience of clinicians. Fearing that three hours of painstaking exposition of RCT data had just been flushed down a toilet, and perhaps angry about such dismissal of years of daily effort by researchers like me, I wanted to retort: "Only if you don't care about science." But a debate about philosophy of science could not occur then and there.

This is the problem: yes, statistics do not tell you what to do with the individual case, but this does not mean that a clinician should decide what to do out of thin air. The clinician's decisions about the individual case need to be *informed*, not *dictated*, by scientific knowledge as established in a general way through statistics.

This insight is present in the great neo-Hippocratic thinkers of modern medicine. Perhaps the best example is William Osler, who always emphasized that medicine was not just a science, but also an art, and that the art of medicine is the art of balancing probabilities (Osler, 1932). If we use the reality of art to negate the necessity of science, we might as well start Galenic bleeding all over again. The art of medicine is, as Osler suggests, in fact, the proper appreciation of the science via a knowledge of statistics: *the art of balancing probabilities*.

The problem with that colleague's comment was that he was *negating* the general knowledge of statistics by prioritizing the individual experience of clinicians. The history of medicine, and a rational approach to the philosophy of science, indicates that the prioritization should be the other way around (which is the basic perspective of EBM).

The illogic of hypothesis-testing statistics

When most people use the word "logic," they mean what philosophers call "predicate" logic, meaning discussions of statements about present facts: things that *are*. However, what may be true in *predicate* logic – things that *are* – may not be true for other kinds of logic, such as *modal* logic – things that *possibly or probably* are. As noted in Chapter 7, Jacob Cohen's intuition (Cohen, 1994), translated into the language of logic, is that the key problem with hypothesis-testing statistics is that *it works in predicate logic, but fails in modal logic*.

Logic is important. As a branch of philosophy, it examines whether one's conclusions flow from one's premises. Logic is an important method, because no matter what the content of one's views, if the logical structure of an argument is invalid, then the whole argument is faulty. We may or may not agree with the content of any statement (the world is round; the world is flat), but we should all be able to agree on the logic of any claim that if X is true, then Y must be true. If an argument is illogical, then it can simply be dismissed.

Now let's see why hypothesis-testing statistics is illogical. Predicate logic applied to hypothesis-testing statistics would be as follows:

> If the null hypothesis [NH] is correct, then these data *cannot occur*.
> These data have occurred.
> Therefore, the null hypothesis *is false*.

This argument is logically valid; but it becomes invalid once it is turned into a statement of probability:

> If the null hypothesis [NH] is correct, then these data *are highly unlikely*.
> These data have occurred.
> Therefore, the null hypothesis *is highly unlikely*.

I have italicized the differences where we have moved from statements of fact to statements of probability. The falsity of this transition becomes clear once we use examples. Using predicate logic:

> If a person is a Martian, then he/she is not a member of Congress.
> This person is a member of Congress.
> Therefore, he/she is not a Martian.

This logic of facts is valid; but the logic of probability is invalid:

> If a person is an American then he is probably not a member of Congress.
> This person is a member of Congress.
> Therefore, he is probably not American.
>
> (Pollard and Richardson, 1987)

Cohen calls this logical fallacy "the illusion of attaining improbability," and if true, which appears to be the case, it undercuts the very basis of hypothesis-testing statistics, and thereby, the vast majority of medical research. The whole industry of p-values comes tumbling down.

Inductive logic

Medical statistics are based on observation, and thus they are a species of induction. Induction, in turn, is philosophically complex. It turns out that one cannot easily infer causation from observation, and that the logic of our hypothesis-testing methods is faulty. What are we to do?

Once again, the answer seems to be to give up our theories and return more closely to our observation. The more we engage in descriptive statistics, the farther away we get from hypothesis-mongering, the closer we are to a conceptually sound use of statistics. We can quantitate without over-speculating.

I hope some day to be able to publish research studies on small sample sizes where the results can be accepted as they are, with the main limitation of imprecision, but without the irrelevant claim that they can only be "hypothesis-generating" as opposed to "hypothesis-testing." Science is not about hypothesis-testing or hypothesis-generating; it is about the complex interrelation between theory and fact, and the gradual accumulation of evidence for or against any scientific hypothesis. Perhaps we can then get beyond the logical fallacies so rampant in statistical debates, so closely related to the lament of a philosopher: "All logic texts are divided into two parts. In the first part, on deductive logic, the fallacies are explained; in the second part, on inductive logic, they are committed." (Cohen, 1994.)

The limits of statistics

Evidence-based medicine: defense and criticism

> Statistics are curious things. They afford one of the few examples in which the use, or abuse, of mathematical methods tends to induce a strong emotional reaction in non-mathematical minds.
>
> Austin Bradford Hill (Hill, 1971; p. vii)

There is a case to be made for evidence-based medicine (EBM), and there is a case to be made against it. Many of the critiques of EBM are, I believe, ill-founded; but there are some important criticisms that need attention. Recently, for example, prominent biologically oriented senior figures in psychiatry have published provocative papers in critique of EBM as applied to psychiatry (Levine and Fink, 2006). They argue that EBM can only be applied to psychiatry if three assumptions hold: "Is the diagnostic system valid? Are the data from clinical trials assessing efficacy and safety valid? Are they in a form that can be applied to clinical practice?" The authors then conclude negatively on all three fronts, high-lighting the limitations of the DSM-IV psychiatric nosology, referring to misconduct in the practice of clinical trials (e.g., inclusion of borderline qualifying patients), and emphasizing how the pharmaceutical industry misuses clinical trials for its own economic purposes. Others have appropriately emphasized the importance of the humanities, as opposed to just EBM, in psychiatry (Bolwig, 2006). And still others note the persistence of authority ("eminence-based medicine") as a key aspect of psychiatric practice, suggesting that EBM cannot replace it (Stahl, 2002). Despite some attempts in the psychiatric literature (Soldani *et al.*, 2005) to clarify the uses of EBM, as well as its limits, there still seems to be a mistrust about the EBM approach among many psychiatrists.

Here I will make the case for EBM, and then we can see its limitations. The context I will use relates to psychiatry, but most of the same issues apply to all of medicine.

The history of non-EBM

Evidence-based medicine as a name and a movement is only a few decades old; but as a concept it is ancient, and thus to appreciate it, one must begin long ago.

In the fifth century AD, a brilliant physician had a powerful idea: the four humors, in varied combinations, produced all illness. From that date until a century ago, Galen's theory ruled medicine. Its corollary was that the treatment of disease involved getting the humors back in order; releasing them through bloodletting was the most common procedure, often augmented by other means of freeing bodily fluids (e.g., purgatives and laxatives). For 14 centuries, physicians subscribed to this wondrous biological theory of disease: we bled our patients until they lost their entire blood supply; we forced them to puke and defecate and urinate; we alternated extremely hot showers with extremely frigid ones – all in the name of normalizing those humors (Porter, 1997). It all proved to be wrong.

This is not a "Whiggish" (or progressive) interpretation of history: it is not simply a matter of "they were wrong and we are right." Galen, Avicenna, Benjamin Rush – these were far more intelligent and creative men than we are. Not only am I not Whiggish, I believe we are repeating these past errors: 14 centuries of ignorance have sunk deep marks into the flesh of the medical profession. As Sir George Pickering, Regius Professor of Medicine at Oxford, said in 1949: "Modern medicine still preserves much of the attitude of mind of the schoolmen of the Middle Ages. It tends to be omniscient rather than admit ignorance, to encourage speculation not solidly backed by evidence, and to be indifferent to the proof or disproof of hypothesis. It is to this legacy of the Middle Ages that may be attributed the phenomenon . . . (of) 'the mysterious viability of the false.'" (Hill, 1962; p. 176.)

We see this influence even today in such articles as the aforementioned critique of EBM as applied to psychiatry. I will be repeating some notions described in other chapters, but this repetition is meant to solidify in the reader's mind the importance of such concepts. Let us review the scientific and conceptual rationale for statistics in general, and for EBM in particular.

Galen versus Hippocrates

There are, and always have been, two basic philosophies of medicine. One is *Galenic*: there is a theory, and it is right. For our purposes, the content of such theories do not matter (they can be about humors, serotonin and dopamine neurotransmitters (Stahl, 2005), ECT (Fink and Taylor, 2007), or even psychoanalysis): what matters is that hardly any scientific theory (especially in medicine) is absolutely right (Ghaemi, 2003). The error is not so much in the content, but in the method of this way of thinking: the focus is on theory, not reality; on beliefs, not facts; on concepts, not clinical observations. If the facts do not agree with the theory, so much the worse for the facts. This perspective led Galen to think that if patients did not respond to his treatments, they were *ipso facto* incurable (shades of notions like "treatment-resistant depression"):

> All who drink of this treatment recover in a short time,
> Except those whom it does not help, who all die.
> It is obvious, therefore, that it fails only in incurable cases.
>
> Galen (Silverman, 1998; p. 3)

There is, and has always been, a second approach, much more humble and simple – the idea that clinical observation, first and foremost, should precede any theory; that theories should be sacrificed to observations, and not vice versa; and clinical realities are more basic than any other theory. This second approach was first propulgated clearly by *Hippocrates* and his school in the fifth century BC, but Galen demolished Hippocratic medicine (while claiming its mantle) and it lay dormant until revived 1000 years later in the Renaissance (McHugh, 1996; Ghaemi, 2008).

Hippocratic humility

Why all this historical background in a discussion of EBM? Because it is important to know what the options, and what the stakes, are. Either we are Hippocratic or we are Galenic; either we value clinical observation or we value theories. The debate comes down to this.

If readers, including EBM critics, claim that they value clinical observation, then the question is: how can we validate clinical observation? How do we know when our observations are correct and when they are false?

Readers of this book will recognize that the core problem is *confounding bias* (Miettinen and Cook, 1981); a deep and very basic clinical problem: *we, clinicians, cannot believe our eyes*. It can appear that something is the case, when it is not; that some treatment is improving matters, when it is not. These confounding factors are present not just some of the time, but *most* of the time.

Now perhaps most clinicians would admit this basic fact, but it is important to draw both the *clinical* and *scientific* implications.

Clinically, the reality of confounding bias teaches us the deep need for a Hippocratic humility, as opposed to a Galenic arrogance – a recognition that we might be wrong, indeed we often are, even in our most definitive clinical experiences (Ghaemi, 2008). Everybody thought Galen was right for 14 centuries; the end of Galenic treatments came about in the nineteenth century *because of* EBM – "the numerical method" of Pierre Louis (Porter, 1997). *Counting patients*, the numerical method, EBM – that has been the source of the greatest medical advances, not the exquisite case study, nor the brilliance of any person (be he/she Freud or Kraepelin or even our most prominent professors today), nor decades of clinical experience. Hill noted that the common distinction between clinical experience and clinical research is a false one (Hill, 1962): after all, clinical experience is based on the recollection of cases, usually a few cases; clinical research is simply the claim that such recollection is biased, and that the remedy is to collect more than just a few cases, *and* to compare them in ways that reduce bias. The latter point entails EBM.

Truths of theory are transient. Not only is Galen out of date, but so is the much vaunted catecholamine theory of depression; today's most sophisticated neurobiology will be passé by the end of the decade. Clinical observation and research, in contrast, is more steady: that same melancholia that Hippocrates described can be discerned in today's major depression; that same mania that Arateus of Cappadocia explained in the second century AD is visible in current mania. (Obviously social and cultural factors come into play, and such presentations vary somewhat in different epochs, as social constructionists will point out [Foucault, 1994].) Clinical research is the solid ground of medicine; biological theory is a necessary but changing superstructure. If these relations are reversed, then mere speculation takes over, and the more solid ground of science is lost.

Scientifically, confounding bias leads to the conclusion that *any* observation, even the most repeated and detailed, can be – indeed often is – wrong; thus valid clinical judgments can only be made after removing confounding factors (Miettinen and Cook, 1981; Rothman and Greenland, 1998).

Randomization, as discussed throughout this book, is the most effective way to remove confounding bias, and it has disproven many widely accepted treatments that proved to be ineffective, harmful, or both.

If we accept, then, that clinical observation is the core of medicine (rather than theory), and that confounding bias afflicts it, and that randomization is the best solution, then we have accepted EBM. That is the core of EBM, and the rationale for the levels of evidence where randomized data are more valid than observational data (Soldani *et al.*, 2005). These are new methods and major advances in medical treatment in the past 50 years are unimaginable without randomized clinical trials (RCTs) in specific, and EBM in general. Indeed, perhaps the greatest public health advance of our era – the linking of cigarette smoking and cancer (led by Hill) – was both source and consequence of EBM methods. As to the relevance of EBM to psychiatry, after the streptomycin RCT (Hill, 1971), among the first RCTs to happen were in psychiatry: with chlorpromazine and lithium in the early 1950s (Healy, 2001).

Psychiatric nosology

Critics of EBM often make much of the limitations of psychiatric nosology (Levine and Fink, 2006). Yet EBM has little to do with diagnosis. Evidence-based medicine, as formally advanced in recent years (Sackett *et al.*, 2000), has mainly had to do with treatment, not diagnosis; it focuses on treatment studies, on randomization (which is only relevant to treatment, not diagnosis), and on such statistical techniques that relate to treatment (such as meta-analysis, number needed to treat, etc.) (Sackett *et al.*, 2000). Validating diagnoses is a matter for another field (clinical epidemiology) (Robins and Guze, 1970; Ghaemi, 2003). (To the extent that diagnosis is addressed at all in most of the EBM literature, it has to do with subjects such as the sensitivity and specificity of diagnostic tests, the classic example being V/Q scans for deep venous thrombosis (Jaeschke *et al.*, 1994), not theoretical questions about etiology of illnesses or diagnostic criteria.) One could define schizophrenia in a completely opposite manner as DSM-IV does; assessments of treatment would still need to account for confounding bias, and the consequent validity of RCTs would still hold.

One can be, not unjustifiably, fed up with DSM-IV and its impact on contemporary psychiatry; but there is no rationale in blaming EBM for it. We are dealing with the true (DSM-IV has many faults), true (EBM has limitations), and unrelated (they have nothing to do with each other).

The pharmaceutical industry

The same holds for critiques of how RCTs are designed and conducted and influences of the pharmaceutical industry. None of this gets at the core rationale for EBM. Indeed, for-profit research groups can conduct clinical research invalidly and unethically, as can pharmaceutical companies; but the same could be said about the private practice of medicine, which can be conducted unethically and yet does not invalidate clinical medicine as such. Evidence-based medicine is not invalidated based on details about how clinical trials are run; randomized trials can still be faulty for many reasons (dropouts can be high, inclusion and exclusion criteria can be wrong, and so on) (Friedman *et al.*, 1998). But again this only means that those studies need to be conducted correctly, not incorrectly. The core rationale for randomized clinical trials (to remove confounding bias) remains unaffected.

Anti-statistics bias

There is, I believe, a general anti-statistics bias among many critics of EBM, and this bias has existed since the 1800s, from the first attempts of Pierre Louis or Quetelet to apply statistics to any human activity. Some critics seem to have an unconscious libertarian streak, as if statistics removes the soul from humanity and deprives individuals of free will. Others come at the issue from a Galenic view of medicine, as if biological theories should trump clinical observations, or, alternatively, clinical observations alone – a statistical accumulation of numbers – are meaningless if not biologically explained. (These critics call this the "medical," as opposed to the statistical, approach to EBM.) (Fink and Taylor, 2008.)

These critics would do well to re-examine that primal medical controversy: cigarette smoking and lung cancer. As discussed previously (Chapter 10), the importance of medical statistics grew out of, and was proven by, this controversy. This is now a matter that has been well documented historically (Parascandola, 2004). Medicine, like politics, involves a great deal of moral responsibility, because human lives are in play. How many lives were lost over half a century of indecision, partly due to an ill-informed attack on statistics by biologically oriented physicians? Critics of EBM need to keep this history in mind.

The cult of the Swan-Ganz catheter

Nor need one go back far in history. We have good examples today of the hazards of this apparently hard-nosed "biological" approach to medicine, disparaging clinical research and statistical methods. A great example is the Swan-Ganz catheter, a staple of coronary intensive care units throughout the 1980s and 1990s. I recall, as a medical intern in 1990, how much ritual was involved with the use of the Swan: dialing some of the treatments up, others down, getting moment-by-moment blood pressure readings. It all seemed as scientific as one could possibly be. But it was all untested by clinical research methods, and, now disproven by RCTs, it has proven to be a farce, and a deadly one, since the placement of the catheter in the neck was a complicated and dangerous procedure. Despite a warning article in 1985 by a medical leader, called "The cult of the Swan-Ganz catheter" (Robin, 1985), clinicians went along aggressively using it. As one physician describes now, looking back: "Those of us in the cult of the Swan-Ganz catheter had many motivations to join: true belief based on experience or (less likely) research studies, economic interest, a desire to give our patients what is now called 'standard of care,' frustration at our lack of effective treatments, the need to feel that we were helping, the need to impress our attendings, or laziness." (Blank, 2006.) Without EBM, all of medicine approximates a cult, with charismatic leaders and passionate followers. The dangers of a cult of medicine, however, are that not only are minds at risk, but so are bodies.

Ivory-tower EBM

This is my defense of EBM, but I believe it deserves criticism as well, just different critiques than those raised above.

I think the most important but underappreciated misuse is what might be called *ivory-tower EBM* – the idea that unless there are double-blind randomized placebo-controlled data, then there *is* no "evidence" (Soldani *et al.*, 2005). But there is always evidence: that is the whole point of EBM, to give us a method whereby we can weigh that evidence. Even non-randomized evidence may be correct and useful (in the absence of randomized data or given certain constraints; for instance the link between cigarettes and smoking is completely based on non-randomized evidence, but with a great deal of careful statistical analysis to assess confounding factors). This view reflects a rarefied positivism that reflects a lack of understanding of the nature of evidence (and science) (Soldani *et al.*, 2005). In my experience as a researcher and author, it is not uncommon to hear academic leaders (and journal peer reviewers) disparage important observational data as mere "chart reviews," as if they are thereby useless. This is the dogma of the cost-cutters, whether they be insurance companies or even national governments. This kind of fetishization of RCTs reflects a misunderstanding of science. We need informed critiques of EBM – because it can be misunderstood, and even abused – not to destroy, but rather to improve it.

Back to Galen

It is an irony of history, but the whole development of medical statistics can be seen as an attempt to end the Galenic tyranny of theory, an effort to end medical dogmatism, a wish to exalt the simple virtues of Hippocratic observation. Ivory-tower EBM brings us back to Galen, the purveyor of medical dogmatism, the ogre which Louis and Fisher and Hill had tried to slay through the development of medical statistics. Now, ironically, the peak of statistical activism, EBM run amuck, threatens to bring back the sacrifice of observations to theory.

The medical epidemiologist Alvan Feinstein (Feinstein and Horwitz, 1997) emphasizes the problem of the "average patient," the fact that RCTs produce average results for a homogeneous sample, rather than showing effects in clinically relevant subtypes. The clinician treats an old man, or a young girl, but the average of those two persons is a middle-aged hermaphrodite. The clinical trial, even if valid internally, just does not directly generalize to the individual patient seen by a clinician. This problem goes beyond generalizability, and brings us back to the conceptual problem of the individual versus the general, as discussed in Chapter 11. The fetishization of RCTs reaches its climax, he argued, in the Cochrane Collaboration, the "industrial scale" application of meta-analysis to determine the "best" available evidence (see Chapter 13). The Cochrane database completely ignores all observational studies, and thus it would not include any "evidence" that penicillin is effective. Hence any attempt to claim "authoritative evidence," especially a methodology that would ignore penicillin, should raise our suspicion, Feinstein concludes. Such authoritarian claims, especially when manipulated in meta-analysis, can easily be abused, and "a new form of dogmatic authoritarianism may then be revived in modern medicine, but the pronouncements will come from Cochranian Oxford rather than Galenic Rome." (Feinstein and Horwitz, 1997.)

Parachutes for gravitational challenge

A. Bradford Hill noted that RCTs were unnecessary in certain cases; sometimes the effect of a treatment is so massive that its benefits are obvious: an example is penicillin. Sometimes, the disease is invariably fatal, so any benefit seen can be taken as real; Hill used the example of miliary or meningeal tuberculosis, invariably fatal conditions in contrast to pulmonary tuberculosis, which has a variable course. It is precisely in such variable conditions, Hill argued, that RCTs are needed. He was able to convince British authorities to allow the 1948 RCT of streptomycin for pulmonary, but not miliary or meningeal, tuberculosis on this rationale (Silverman, 1998; pp. 98–100).

Many proponents of ivory-tower EBM do not appreciate Hill's insight: RCTs are not needed when outcomes are invariable.

This reality, so obvious to common sense but opaque to those who have become EBM true believers, was acknowledged by the *British Journal of Medicine*, which published a tongue-in-cheek article (written by obstetricians at Cambridge University in the UK) entitled: "Parachute use to prevent death and major trauma related to gravitational challenge: systematic review of randomized, controlled trials" (Smith and Pell, 2003). The authors reported, after searching "Medline, Web of Science, Embase, and the Cochrane library databases": "We were unable to identify any randomized controlled trials of parachute intervention." They noted that "the basis for parachute use is purely observational," and that the role of bias could not be discounted because "individuals jumping from aircraft without the help of a parachute are likely to have a high prevalence of pre-existing psychiatric morbidity and may also differ in key demographic factors, such as income and cigarette use. It follows, therefore, that the apparent protective effect of parachutes may be merely an example of the 'healthy cohort' effect." They noted that no "multivariate analytical approaches" had tried to correct for these biases. They also decried that the use of parachutes was just another example of disease-mongering (see Chapter 17), "the medicalisation of free fall": "It might be argued that the pressure exerted on individuals to use parachutes is yet another example of a natural, life enhancing experience being turned into a situation of fear and dependency." Economic factors could not be ignored (see Chapter 17): "The parachute industry has earned billions of dollars for vast multinational corporations whose profits depend on belief in the efficacy of their product. One would hardly expect these vast commercial concerns to have the bravery to test their product in the setting of a randomized controlled trial." They conclude: "Individuals who insist that all interventions need to be validated by a randomized controlled trial need to come down to earth with a bump." (Smith and Pell, 2003.)

"The world is round (p < 0.05)"

Another way of looking at the limitations of EBM is to realize that EBM is less applicable where quantitative methods are irrelevant or inapplicable. The statistician Jacob Cohen emphasized the limitations of medical statistics, the basis for EBM, with the above title to one of his papers (Cohen, 1994).

As described in Chapter 11, the work of science is not about definitively proving or disproving any theory with any single study. "Facts" do not exist separate from theories, and thus scientific hypotheses are always only partially proven or disproven with specific studies. The convergence of replicated research, gradually approximating the truth (as Peirce [1958] described), is how science works. No p-value, and no RCT (and no meta-analysis), captures that convergence. For a long time, the world's consensus was that the world is flat. Over time, the consensus changed to the world being round. There are good grounds for this change, but they have nothing to do with p-values.

Appreciating, not abusing, EBM

Those who think EBM cannot be applied to psychiatry or medicine should think about the implications given the history of medicine. Without the application of scientific principles to clinical research, we will have nothing but opinion – a postmodern relativist world where all is ideology. Without scientific, evidence-based clinical research, in the Hippocratic tradition of careful attention to clinical observation – and its statistical correlates in the need for combating confounding bias – psychiatry, and all of medicine, would be but a mere shadow of what is, and a pale reflection of what it can be. Not only should EBM be applied to psychiatry, but, if we do not, we will just go back to the brackish dogmatisms of the past, a return to a non-Hippocratic approach to medicine which failed humanity for so long. Two millennia are long enough to test a theory.

On the other hand, let us not make a fetish out of RCTs. Recall cigarettes once more: many important features of human disease cannot be settled by RCTs. Evidence-based medicine means *levels* of evidence, and a recognition of the *limits* of statistics (as well as their uses); not an ivory-tower positivism, an idealization of all-powerful placebo-based data, standing as absolute Truth; not a tool to be used for political or economic purposes, a fetish of governments, a profit-making plan for insurance companies, and a marketing mechanism for pharmaceutical companies. Evidence-based medicine, properly understood, should be a scientific tool for applying medical statistics to clinical practice. But using such a tool implies understanding the limitations of both medical statistics and clinical practice.

13 The alchemy of meta-analysis

> Exercising the right of occasional suppression and slight modification, it is truly
> absurd to see how plastic a limited number of observations become, in the hands of
> men with preconceived ideas.
>
> Sir Francis Galton, 1863 (Stigler, 1986; p. 267)

It is an interesting fact that meta-analysis is the product of psychiatry. It was developed specifically to refute a critique, made in the 1960s by the irrepressible psychologist Hans Eysenck, that psychotherapies (mainly psychoanalytic) were ineffective (Hunt, 1997). Yet the word "meta-analysis" seems too awe-inspiring for most mental health professionals to even begin to approach it. This need not be the case.

The rationale for meta-analysis is to provide some systematic way of putting together all the scientific literature on a specific topic. Though Eysenck was correct that there are many limitations to meta-analysis, we cannot avoid the fact that we will always be trying to make sense of the scientific literature as a whole, and not just study by study. If we don't use meta-analysis methods, we will inevitably be using some methods to make these judgments, most of which have even more faults than meta-analysis. In Chapter 14, we will also see another totally different mindset, Bayesian statistics, as a way to put all the knowledge base together for clinical practice.

Critics have noted that meta-analysis resembles alchemy (Feinstein, 1995), taking the dross of individually negative studies to produce the gold of a positive pooled result. But alchemy led to the science of chemistry, and properly used, meta-analysis can advance our knowledge.

So let us see what meta-analysis is all about, and how it fares compared to other ways of reviewing the scientific literature.

Non-systematic reviews

There is likely to be broad consensus that the least acceptable approach to a review of the literature is the classic "selective" review, in which the reviewer selects those articles which agree with his opinion, and ignores those which do not. On this approach, any opinion can be supported by selectively choosing among studies in the literature. The opposite of the selective review is the systematic review. In this approach, some effort is made, usually with computerized searching, to identify all studies on a topic. Once all studies are identified (including ideally some that may not have been published), then the question is how these studies can be compared.

The simplest approach to reviewing a literature is the "vote count" method: how many studies were positive, how many negative? The problem with this approach is that it fails to take into account the quality of the various studies (i.e., sample sizes, randomized or not, control of bias, adequacy of statistical testing for chance). The next most rigorous approach is a pooled analysis. This approach corrects for sample size, unlike vote counting, but nothing else. Other features of studies are not assessed, such as bias in design, randomization or not, and so on. Sometimes, those features can be controlled by inclusion criteria which might, for instance, limit a pooled analysis to only randomized studies.

Meta-analysis defined

Meta-analysis represents an *observational study of studies*. In other words, one tries to combine the results of many different studies into one summary measure. This is, to some extent, unavoidable in that clinicians and researchers need to try to pull together different studies into some useful summary of the state of the literature on a topic. There are different ways to go about this, with meta-analysis perhaps the most useful, but all reviews also have their limitations.

Apples and oranges

Meta-analysis weights studies by their samples sizes, but in addition, meta-analysis corrects for the variability of the data (some studies have smaller standard deviations, and thus their results are more precise and reliable). The problem still remains that studies differ from each other, the problem of "heterogeneity" (sometimes called the "apples and oranges" problem), which reintroduces confounding bias when the actual results are combined. The main attempts to deal with this problem in meta-analysis are the same as in observational studies. (Randomization is not an option because one cannot randomize studies, only patients within a study.) One option is to exclude certain confounding factors through strict inclusion criteria. For instance, a meta-analysis may only include women, and thus gender is not a confounder; or perhaps a meta-analysis would be limited to the elderly, thus excluding confounding by younger age. Often, meta-analyses are limited to randomized clinical trials (RCTs) only, as in the Cochrane Collaboration, with the idea being that patient samples will be less heterogeneous in the highly controlled setting of RCTs as opposed to observational studies. Nonetheless, given that meta-analysis itself is an observational study, it is important to realize that the benefits of randomization are lost. Often readers may not realize this point, and thus it may seem that a meta-analysis of ten RCTs is more meaningful than each RCT alone. However, each large well-conducted RCT is basically free of confounding bias, while no meta-analysis is completely free of confounding bias. The most meaningful findings are when individual RCTs and the overall meta-analysis all point in the same direction.

Another way to handle the confounding bias of meta-analysis, just as in single observational studies, is to use stratification or regression models, often called meta-regression. For instance, if ten RCTs exist, but five used crossover design and five used parallel design, one could create a regression model in which the relative risk of benefit with drug versus placebo is obtained corrected for variables of crossover design and parallel design. Meta-regression methods are relatively new.

Publication bias

Besides the apples and oranges problem, the other major problem of meta-analysis is the publication bias, or file-drawer, problem. The issue here is that the published literature may not be a valid reflection of the reality of research on a topic because positive studies are more often published than negative studies. This occurs for various reasons. Editors may be more inclined to reject negative studies given the limits of publication space. Researchers may be less inclined to put effort into writing and revising manuscripts of negative studies given the lack of interest engendered by such reports. And, perhaps most importantly, pharmaceutical companies who conduct RCTs have a strong economic motivation *not* to publish negative studies of their drugs. When published, their competitors would likely seize upon negative findings to attack a company's drug, and the cost of preparing and producing such manuscripts would likely be hard to justify to the marketing managers of a for-profit company. In summary, there are many reasons that lead to the systematic suppression of negative treatment studies. Meta-analyses would then be biased toward positive findings for efficacy of treatments. One possible way around this problem, which has gradually begun to be implemented, is to create a data registry where all RCTs conducted on a topic would be registered. If studies were not published, then managers of those registries would obtain the actual data from negative studies and store them for the use of systematic reviews and meta-analyses. This possible solution is limited by the fact that it is dependent on the voluntary cooperation of researchers, and in the case of the pharmaceutical industry, with a few exceptions, most companies refuse to provide such negative data (Ghaemi *et al.*, 2008a). The patent and privacy laws in the US protect them on this issue, but this factor makes definitive scientific reviews of evidence difficult to achieve.

Clinical example: meta-analysis of antidepressants in bipolar depression

Recently, the first meta-analysis of antidepressant use in acute bipolar depression identified only five placebo-controlled studies in the literature (Gijsman *et al.*, 2004). The conclusion of the meta-analysis was that antidepressants were more effective than placebo for acute depression, and that they had not been shown to cause more manic switch than placebo. However, important issues of heterogeneity were not explored. For instance, the only placebo-controlled study which found no evidence of acute antidepressant response is the only study (Nemeroff *et al.*, 2001) where all patients received baseline lithium. Among other studies, one (Cohn *et al.*, 1989) non-randomly assigned 37% of patients in the antidepressant arm to lithium versus 21% in the placebo arm: a relative 77% increased lithium use in the antidepressant arm, hardly a fair assessment of fluoxetine versus placebo. Two compared antidepressant alone to placebo alone and one large study (Tohen *et al.*, 2003) (58.5% of all meta-analysis patients), compared olanzapine plus fluoxetine to olanzapine alone ("placebo" improperly refers to olanzapine plus placebo). These studies may suggest acute antidepressant efficacy compared to no treatment or olanzapine alone, but not compared to the most proven mood stabilizer, lithium, which is also the most relevant clinical issue.

Regarding antidepressant-induced mania, two studies comparing antidepressants without mood stabilizer to no treatment (placebo only) report no mania in any patients: an oddity, if true, since it would suggest that even spontaneous mania did not occur while those patients were studied, or that perhaps manic symptoms were not adequately assessed. As described above, another study preferentially prescribed lithium more in the antidepressant group (Cohn *et al.*, 1989), providing possibly unequal protection against mania. While the olanzapine/fluoxetine data suggest no evidence of switch while using antipsychotics, notably in our reanalysis of the lithium plus paroxetine (or imipramine) study, there was a threefold higher manic switch rate with imipramine versus placebo (risk ratio 3.14), with asymmetrically positively skewed confidence intervals (0.34, 29.0). These studies were not powered to assess antidepressant-induced mania, and thus lack of a finding is liable to type II false negative error. It is more effective to use descriptive statistics as above, which suggest some likelihood of higher manic switch risk at least with tricyclic antidepressants (TCAs) compared to placebo.

Thus, apparent agreement among studies hides major conflicting results between the only adequately designed study using the most proven mood stabilizer, lithium, and the rest (either no mood stabilizer use or use of less proven agents).

Meta-analysis as interpretation

The above example demonstrates the dangers of meta-analysis, as well as some of its benefits. Ultimately, meta-analysis is not the simple quantitative exercise that it may appear to be, and that some of its aficionados appear to believe is the case. It involves many, many interpretive judgments, much more than in the usual application of statistical concepts to a single clinical trial. Its real danger, then, as Eysenck tried to emphasize (Eysenck, 1994), is that it can put an *end* to discussion, based on biased interpretations cloaked with quantitative authority, rather than leading to more accurate evaluation of available studies. At root, Eysenck points out that what matters is the *quality* of the studies, a matter that is not itself a quantitative question (Eysenck, 1994).

Meta-analysis can clarify, and it can obfuscate. By choosing one's inclusion and exclusion criteria carefully, one can still prove whatever point one wishes. Sometimes meta-analyses of the same topic, published by different researchers, directly conflict with each other. Meta-analysis is a tool, not an answer. We should not let this method control us, doing meta-analyses willy-nilly on any and all topics (as unfortunately appears to be the habit of some researchers), but rather cautiously and selectively where the evidence seems amenable to this kind of methodology.

Meta-analysis is less valid than RCTs

One last point deserves to be re-emphasized, a point which meta-analysis mavens sometimes dispute, without justification: *meta-analysis is never more valid than an equally large single RCT*. This is because a single RCT of 500 patients means that the whole sample is randomized and confounding bias should be minimal. But a meta-analysis of 5 different RCTs that add up to a total of 500 patients is *no longer a randomized study*. Meta-analysis is an observational pooling of data; the fact that the data were originally randomized no longer applies once they are pooled. So if they conflict, the results of meta-analysis, despite the fanciness of the word, should never be privileged over a large RCT. In the case of the example above, that methodologically flawed meta-analysis does not come close to the validity of a recently published large RCT of 366 patients randomized to antidepressants versus placebo for bipolar depression, in which, contrary to the meta-analysis, there was no benefit with antidepressants (Sachs *et al.*, 2007).

Statistical alchemy

Alvan Feinstein (Feinstein, 1995) has thoughtfully critiqued meta-analysis in a way that pulls together much of the above discussion. He notes that, after much effort, scientists have come to a consensus about the nature of science; it must have four features: reproducibility, "precise characterization," unbiased comparisons ("internal validity"), and appropriate generalization ("external validity"). Readers will note that he thereby covers the same territory I use in this book as the three organizing principles of statistics: bias, chance, and causation. Meta-analysis, Feinstein argues, ruins all this effort. It does so because it seeks to "convert existing things into something better. 'Significance' can be attained statistically when small group sizes are pooled into big ones; and new scientific hypotheses, that had inconclusive results or that had not been originally tested, can be examined for special subgroups or other entities." These benefits come at the cost, though, of "the removal or destruction of the scientific requirements that have been so carefully developed …"

He makes the analogy to alchemy because of "the idea of getting something for nothing, while simultaneously ignoring established scientific principles." He calls this the "free lunch" principle, which makes meta-analysis suspect, along with the "mixed salad" principle, his metaphor for heterogeneity (implying even more drastic differences than apples and oranges).

He notes that meta-analysis violates one of Hill's concepts of causation: the notion of *consistency*. Hill thought that studies should generally find the same result; meta-analysis accepts studies with differing results, and privileges some over others: "With meta-analytic aggregates … the important inconsistencies are ignored and buried in the statistical agglomeration."

Perhaps most importantly, Feinstein worried that researchers would stop doing better and better studies, and spend all their time trying to wrench truth from meta-analysis of poorly done studies. In effect, meta-analysis is unnecessary where it is valid, and unhelpful where it is needed: where studies are poorly done, meta-analysis is unhelpful, only combining highly heterogeneous and faulty data, thereby producing falsely precise but invalid meta-analytic results. Where studies are well done, meta-analysis is redundant: "My chief complaint … is that meta-analysis of randomized trials concentrates on a part of the scientific domain that is already reasonably well lit, while ignoring the much larger domain that lies either in darkness or in deceptive glitters."

As mentioned in Chapter 12, Feinstein's critique culminates in seeing meta-analysis as a symptom of EBM run amuck (Feinstein and Horwitz, 1997), with the Cochrane Collaboration in Oxford as its symbol, a new potential source of Galenic dogmatism, now in statistical guise. When RCTs are simply immediately put into meta-analysis software, and all other studies are ignored, then the only way in which meta-analysis can be legitimate – careful assessment of quality and attention to heterogeneity – is obviated. Quoting the statistician Richard Peto, Feinstein notes that "the paintstaking detail of a good meta-analysis 'just isn't possible in the Cochrane collaboration' when the procedures are done 'on an industrial scale.'"

Eysenck again

I had the opportunity to meet Eysenck once, and I will never forget his devotion to statistical research. "You cannot have knowledge," he told me over lunch, "unless you can count it." What about the case report, I asked; is that not knowledge at all? He smiled and held up a single finger: "Even then you can count." Eysenck contributed a lot to empirical research in psychology, personality, and psychiatric genetics. Thus, his reservations about meta-analysis are even more relevant, since they do not come from a person averse to statistics, but rather from someone who perhaps knows all too well the limits of statistics.

I will give Eysenck the last word, from a 1994 paper which is among his last writings: "Rutherford once pointed out that when you needed statistics to make your results significant, you would be better off doing a better experiment. Meta-analyses are often used to recover something from poorly designed studies, studies of insufficient statistical power, studies that give erratic results, and those resulting in apparent contradictions. Occasionally, meta-analysis does give worthwhile results, but all too often it is subject to methodological criticisms … Systematic reviews range all the way from highly subjective "traditional" methods to computer-like, completely objective counts of estimates of effect size over all published (and often unpublished) material regardless of quality. Neither extreme seems desirable. There cannot be one best method for fields of study so diverse as those for which meta-analysis has been used. If a medical treatment has an effect so recondite and obscure as to require meta-analysis to establish it, I would not be happy to have it used on me. It would seem better to improve the treatment, and the theory underlying the treatment." (Eysenck, 1994.)

We can summarize. Meta-analysis can be seen as useful in two settings: where research is ongoing, it can be seen as a stop-gap measure, a temporary summary of the state of the evidence, to be superseded by future larger studies. Where further RCT research is uncommon or unlikely, meta-analysis can serve as a more or less definitive summing up of what we know, and thus it can be used to inform Bayesian methods of decision-making.

14 Bayesian statistics: why your opinion counts

> I hope clinicians in the future will abandon the 'margins of the impossible,' and settle for reasonable probability.
>
> Archie Cochrane (Silverman, 1998; p. 37)

Bayesianism is the dirty little secret of statistics. It is the aunt that no one wants to invite to dinner. If mainstream statistics is akin to democratic socialism, Bayesianism often comes across as something like a Trotskyist fringe group, acknowledged at times but rarely tolerated.

Yet, like so many contrarian views, there are probably important truths in this little known and less understood approach to statistics, truths which clinicians in the medical and mental health professions might understand more easily and more objectively than statisticians.

Two philosophies of statistics

There are two basic philosophies of statistics: mainstream current statistics views itself as only assessing data and mathematical interpretations of data – called *frequentist* statistics; the alternative approach sees data as being interpretable only in terms of other data or other probability judgments – this is *Bayesian* statistics. Most statisticians want science to be based on numbers, not opinions, hence, following Fisher, most mainstream statistical methods are frequentist. This frequentist philosophy is not as pure as statisticians might wish, however; throughout this book, I have emphasized the many points in which traditional statistics – and by this I mean the most hard-nosed, data-driven frequentist variety – involves subjective judgments, arbitary cutoffs, and conceptual schemata. This happens not just here and there, but frequently, and in quite important places (two examples are the p-value cutoff and the null hypothesis (NH) definition). But Bayesianism makes subjective judgment part and parcel of the core notion of all statistics: probability. For frequentists, this goes too far. (It might analogize to how capitalists might accept some need for market regulation, but to them socialism seems too extreme.)

In mainstream statistics, the only place where Bayesian concepts are routinely allowed has to do with diagnostic tests (which I will discuss below). More generally, though, there is something special about Bayesian statistics that is worth some effort on the part of clinicians: one might appreciate and even agree with the general wish to base science on hard numbers, not opinions. But clinicians are used to subjectivity and opinions; in fact, much of the instinctive distrust by clinicians of statistics has to do with frequentist assumptions. Bayesian views sit much more comfortably with the unconscious intuitions of clinicians.

Bayes' theorem

There was once a minister, the Reverend Thomas Bayes, who enjoyed mathematics. Living in the mid eighteenth century, Bayes was interested in the early French notions (e.g., Laplace) about probability. Bayes discovered something odd: probabilities appeared to be conditional on something else; they did not exist on their own. So if say that there is a 75% chance that Y will happen, what we are saying is that assuming X, there is a 75% chance that Y will happen. Since X itself is a probability, then we are saying that assuming (let's say) a 80% chance that X will happen, there is a 75% chance that Y will happen. In Bayes' own words, he defines probability thus: "The probability of any event is the ratio between the value at which an expectation depending on the happening of the event ought to be computed, and the value of the thing expected upon its happening." (Bayes and Price, 1763.) The derivation of the mathematical formula – called Bayes' theorem – will not concern us here; suffice it to say that as a matter of mathematics, Bayes' concept is thought to be sound. Stated conceptually, his theorem is that given a prior probability X, the observation of event Y produces a posterior probability Z.

This might be simplified, following Salsburg (Salsburg, 2001; p. 134) as follows:

Prior probability → Data → Posterior probability

Salsburg emphasizes how Bayes' theorem reflects how most humans actually think: "The Bayesian approach is to start with a prior set of probabilities in the mind of a given person. Next, that person observes or experiments and produces data. The data are then used to modify the prior probabilities, producing a posterior set of probabilities." (Salsburg, 2001; p. 134.) Another prominent Bayesian statistician, Donald Berry, put it this way: "Bayes' theorem is a formalism for learning: that's what I thought before, this is what I just saw, so here's what I now think – and I may change my views tomorrow." (Berry, 1993.)

Normally statistics only have to do with Y and Z. We observe certain events Y, and we then infer the probability of that event, or the probability of that event occurring by chance, or some other probability (Z) related to that event. What Bayes adds is an initial probability of the event, a *prior probability*, before we even observe anything. How can this be? And what is this prior probability?

Bayes himself apparently was not sure what to make of the results of his mathematical work. He never published his material, and apparently rarely spoke of it. It came to light after his death and in the nineteenth century had a good deal of influence in the newly developing field of statistics. In the early twentieth century, as the modern foundations of statistics began to be laid by Karl Pearson and Ronald Fisher, however, their first target, and one which they viewed with great animus, was Thomas Bayes.

The attack on Bayes

Bayes' theorem was seen by Pearson and Fisher as dangerous because it introduced *subjectivity* into statistics, and not here and there, or peripherally, but centrally into the very basic concept that underlies all statistics: probability. The prior probability seems suspiciously like simply one's opinion, before observing the data. Pearson and Fisher could agree that if we want statistics to form the basis of modern science, especially in clinical medicine, then we want to base statistics on data and on defensible mathematical formulae that interpret the data, but *not* on simply one's opinion.

The concern has to do with how we establish prior probability: what is it based on? The most obvious answer is that it involves "personal probability." The extreme view, developed by the statistician L. J. Savage is that "there are no such things as proven scientific facts ... There are only statements, about which people who call themselves scientists associate a high probability." (Salsburg, 2001; p. 133.) This is one extreme of Bayesian probability, the most *subjectivist* variety. We might term the other extreme *objectivist*, for it minimizes the subjective opinion of any individual; developed by John Maynard Keynes, the famous economist, this kind of Bayesian probability appeals to me. Keynes' view was that personal probability should not be the view that any person happens to hold, but rather "the degree of belief that an educated person in a given culture can be expected to hold." (Salsburg, 2001; pp. 133–4.) This is similar to Charles Sanders Peirce's view that truth is what the consensus of community of investigators believes to be the case at the limit of scientific investigation. Peirce, like Keynes, was arguing that for scientific concepts in physics, for instance, the opinion of the construction worker does not count the same as the opinion of a professor of physics. What matters is the consensus of those who are of similar background and have similar knowledge base and are engaged in similar efforts to know.

I would take Keynes and Peirce one step further, so as to place Bayesian statistics on even more objective ground, and thus to emphasize to readers that it is valid and, in many ways, not in conflict with standard frequentist statistics. The middle and final terms of Bayes' theorem, as mentioned, are accepted by frequentist mainstream statistics. Data are numbers, not opinions, and certain probabilities can be inferred based on the data. The issue is the prior probability. What if we assert that the prior probability is also solely based on the results of frequentist statistics, i.e., that it is based on the state of the scientific literature? We might use meta-analysis of all available randomized clinical trials (RCTs), for instance, as our prior probability on a given topic. Then a new study would lead to a posterior probability after we incorporate those results with the prior status quo as described in a previous meta-analysis. In that way, the Bayesian structure is used, but with non-subjective and frequentist content. Of course, there will always be some subjectivity to any interpretation, such as meta-analysis, but that level of subjectivity is irremovable and inherent in any kind of statistics, including frequentist methods.

Readers may choose whichever approach they prefer, but I think a case can at least be made for using Bayesian methods with prior probabilities based on the state of the objective scientific literature, and, in doing so, we would not be violating the standards of frequentist mainstream statistics.

Bayesianism in psychiatric practice

Let us pause. Before we reject personal probability as too opinionated, or think of Bayesian approaches as unnecessary or too complex, let me point out that most clinicians – doctors and mental health professionals – operate this way. And accepting personal probability is not equivalent to saying that we must accept a complete relativism about what is probable. Here is an example from a supervision session I recently conducted with a psychiatry resident, Jane, who described a patient of long-standing in our outpatient psychiatry clinic: "No one knows what to do with him," she began. "You won't either, because no one knows the true diagnosis." He was a poor historian and had no family available for corroboration, so important past details of his history could not be obtained. Yet, as she described his history, a few salient points became clear: he had failed to respond to numerous antidepressants for repeated major depressive episodes, which had led to six hospitalizations, beginning at age 22. He had taken all antidepressants, all antipsychotics, and all mood stabilizers. He did not have chronic psychotic symptoms, though possibly had brief such symptoms during his hospitalizations. He had encephalitis at age 17. His family history was unknown. He probably

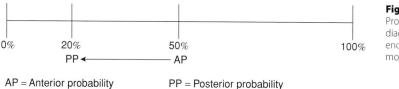

Figure 14.1
Probability of
diagnosis of
encephalitis-induced
mood disorder.

AP = Anterior probability   PP = Posterior probability

had become manic on an antidepressant once, with marked overactivity and hypersexuality just after taking it, compared to no such behavior before or since.

We could only know those facts with reasonable probability. So beginning with the differential diagnosis of recurrent severe depression, I asked her what the possibilities were; quickly it became clear that unipolar depression ("major depressive disorder") was the prime diagnosis; asked about the alternatives, she acknowledged the need to rule out bipolar disorder and secondary mood disorder (depression due to medical illness). Her supposition had been that he had failed to respond to antidepressants for his unipolar depression due to likely concomitant personality disorder, though the nature of that condition was unclear (he did not have classic features of borderline or antisocial personality). Though I acknowledged that possibility, I asked her to think back to the mood disorder differential first.

Let's begin with the conditions that need to be ruled out, I said. The only possible medical illness that could be relevant was encephalitis. Is encephalitis associated with recurrent severe major depressive episodes over two decades later? I asked. We both acknowledged that this was improbable on the basis of the known scientific evidence. So, if we begin with initial complete uncertainty about the role of encephalitis in this recurrent depressive illness, we might start at the 50–50 mark of probability. After consulting the known scientific literature, we then conclude that encephalitis is lower than 50% in probability; if we had to quantify our own personal probability, perhaps it would fall to 20% or less given the absence of any evidence suggesting an encephalitis/long-term recurrent severe depressive illness connection. This is a Bayesian judgment, and can be depicted visually, with 0% reflecting no likelihood of the diagnosis and 100% reflecting absolute certainty of the diagnosis (Figure 14.1).

Next, one could turn to the bipolar disorder differential diagnosis. If we began again with a neutral attitude of complete uncertainty, our anterior probability would be at the 50–50 mark. Beginning to look at the highly probable facts of the clinical history, two facts stand out: antidepressant-induced mania (ADM) and non-response to multiple therapeutic trials of antidepressants (documented in the outpatient records). We can then turn again to known scientific knowledge: ADM occurs in < 1% of persons with unipolar depression, but in 5–50% of persons with bipolar disorder. Thus it is 5- to 50-fold more likely that bipolar disorder is the diagnosis rather than unipolar depression based on that fact. Treatment non-response to three or more adequate antidepressant trials are associated, in some studies, with a 25–50% likelihood of misdiagnosed bipolar disorder, the most common feature associated with such treatment resistance. Thus, both clinical features would make the probability of bipolar disorder higher, not lower. So we would move from the 50% mark closer to the 100% mark. Depending on the strength of the scientific literature, the quality of the studies, the amount of replication, and our own interpretation of that literature, we might move more or less toward 100%, but the direction of movement can only go one way, towards increased probability of diagnosis. If I had to quanitify for myself, I might visually depict it as shown in Figure 14.2.

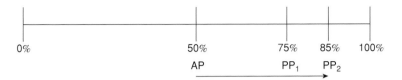

Figure 14.2 Probability of diagnosis of bipolar disorder.

AP = Anterior probability
PP₁ = Posterior probability with ADM.   PP₂ = Posterior probability with ADM + TRD
ADM = antidepressant-induced mania.   TRD = treatment resistant depression

AP = Anterior probability
PP$_1$ = Posterior probability with ADM.   PP$_2$ = Posterior probability with ADM + TRD
ADM = antidepressant-induced mania.   TRD = treatment resistant depression

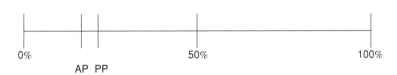

Figure 14.3 Jane's probability of diagnosis of bipolar disorder.

AP = Anterior probability
PP = Posterior probability with ADM + TRD
ADM = antidepressant-induced mania.   TRD = treatment resistant depression

In my personal probability, the likelihood of bipolar disorder increases to the point where it is highly likely. If we assume that at 80% or above likelihood we might make major treatment changes, I might then make major changes in this person's treatment, and insist upon them due to my confidence based on this high level of probability. Now it might be objected that the threshold at which we might change treatments is again subjective, a matter of personal probability, but it is not completely arbitrary: 95% certainty means more than 65% certainty. We can likely agree on a conceptually sound level of certainty, perhaps 80% and above, much as we do in frequentist statistics for concepts such as power or statistical significance.

Once I spelled out this Bayesian rationale for diagnostic probability, my resident Jane was convinced, somewhat against her will. Why had she not reached the same conclusions earlier, and why was she still resistant? Mainly, I believe, it had to do with the sloppy intuitive approach to diagnosis which is so common in clinical practice, combined with the harmful impact of her own assumed biases. In addition, Jane did not know about the studies conducted on ADM and treatment resistant depression (TRD). So there was a problem with lack of factual knowledge, which is usually what methods like evidence-based medicine (EBM) seek to emphasize, but, perhaps more importantly, there was a conceptual problem with unexamined biases. The Bayesian approach brings out these unexamined biases, and thus minimizes them. If we were to depict Jane's Bayesian diagnostic process before we had discussed the case, it would have been something along the lines in Figure 14.3. We start with a low probability of bipolar disorder because she was biased against the diagnosis (in general, it seems; but also most clearly in relation to this patient for whom she intuitively preferred a personality disorder diagnosis). She started out with a very low probability, did not know that TRD would increase it, and felt that ADM would increase it only slightly. Thus, her Bayesian process as regards bipolar disorder might be depictable as in Figure 14.3.

This is her personal probability, but based on the known scientific literature, one cannot plausibly argue that her personal probability was as valid as mine.

Now some readers might say: "wait: you say that she was biased against the bipolar diagnosis, which led her Bayesian reasoning to fail to reach probable levels even with the history

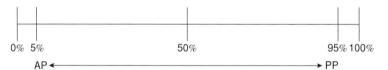

Figure 14.4 The ping-pong effect: frequentist interpretation of conflicting studies.

AP = Anterior probability
PP = Posterior probability

of ADM and TRD. Are not you biased in favor of the bipolar diagnosis? Could not that be why your probabilities ended up closer to 100%?" This would be the case if my anterior initial probability was above 50%. If I had started at 80% probability, then the ADM and TRD features of his illness might take me to 99% as a posterior probability; indeed that might be the case if there was initial bias. But I started at the 50–50 probability level, not higher. This is the neutral point, at which no bias toward any diagnosis is the case. Recall that I also started at 50–50 when assessing the likelihood of encephalitis-induced mood disorder.

If we were to repeat the same Bayesian diagrams with the possible diagnosis of unipolar depression ("major depressive disorder"), we could also begin at the 50–50 level, but we would quickly move, based on the frequentist scientific literature, to a lower probability level due to TRD and ADM.

The main point of this discussion is that the use of Bayesian statistics in this way is not an exercise in completely arbitrary subjectivity. In fact, it decreases our arbitrary, subjective, intuitive approach to clinical practice by forcing us to be explicit about our assumptions and to make at least probabilistic quantifications about them. Further, it relies on the scientific literature, which is based on frequentist methods; it utilizes non-subjective knowledge to inform its subjective probabilistic conclusions (Goodman, 1999).

The ping-pong effect

The two approaches, classical and Bayesian, are based on different conceptual assumptions about the nature of statistical interpretation. Neither approach is definitively right nor wrong. In fact the Bayesian approach not only highlights the limitations of the frequentist approach but it shows why classical frequentist statistics is limited: "Some frequentists talk and write as though they wear glasses that filter out all but null hypotheses. Such an emphasis distorts reality – roughly equivalent to a Bayesian who gives all null hypotheses extremely high prior probability." (Berry, 1993.) Examples of these mainstream statistical blindspots, the author continues, are subgroup analyses and multiple comparisons (discussed in Chapter 8). Most statisticians, being frequentists, err on the side of the NH: unless they are more than 95% certain, they do not consider a finding as notable. This is like, on the visual depictions of diagnostic decision-making above, always starting at the 5% mark, i.e., always having a low prior probability that something is the case. Then if positive data are produced, one would jump to the opposite end and be at the 95% mark, with a very high posterior probability that something is the case. Then again, if the next study is negative, one would jump back to the 5% mark. This ping-pong effect underlies the confusion of many clinicians about opposing results of different scientific studies, depicted in Figure 14.4. If they began in the middle of the visual axis of certainty, however, clinicians would be less liable to be confused, because conflicting data would cancel out and clinicians would throughout remain in the stable state of uncertainty around the 50–50 mark (Figure 14.4).

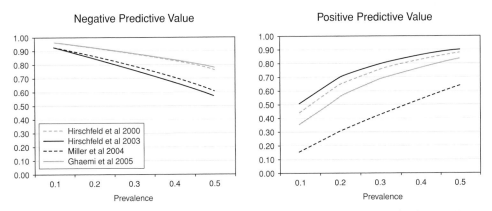

Figure 14.5 Negative versus positive predictive value. From Phelps, J. R. & Ghaemi S. N. (2006) with permission Elsevier. Copyright 2006.

Diagnostic tests

Now I will apply the Bayesian method statistically where it is most clear-cut, in assessing diagnostic screening tests, with my example being patient self-report questionnaires designed to detect bipolar disorder (the Mood Disorders Questionnaire, MDQ; and the Bipolar Spectrum Diagnostic Scale, BSDS). In a study, my colleague Jim Phelps and I applied Bayesian statistical concepts to assess how such a screening tool might be appropriately used, and, in the process, we also saw how classical frequentist statistical assumptions led clinicians and researchers to make grave errors of interpretation (Phelps and Ghaemi, 2006).

Usually those screening tools were reported in terms of the classic frequentist statistics of sensitivity (if the patient has the disease, is the test positive?) and specificity (if the patient does not have the disease, is the test negative?). With high scores on both counts, researchers and clinicians often concluded that positive scores, without any further clinical evaluation, indicated presence of bipolar disorder. Such research was even published in very high-profile scientific journals (Das *et al.*, 2005).

Predictive value, on the other hand, is a Bayesian concept: if the test is positive, how frequently do patients have the disease? (And if negative, how frequently do they not have it?) It turns out that the answer varies, depending on the circumstances, as is the case with Bayesian statistics, unlike classical frequentist statistics: the number does not exist in a vacuum.

Figure 14.5 presents predictive values relative to prevalence, using the sensitivity and specificity data from each of the four studies.

As follows from Bayesian principles, predictive values are inversely affected by prevalence: negative predictive values (NPVs) are high and positive predictive values (PPVs) are low at low prevalence; whereas PPVs are high and NPVs are low at high prevalence. However, PPV is much more sensitive to prevalence than NPV, as manifest in the slope of the respective curves. At low prevalence, which is most relevant to the primary care medicine setting, the sensitivity and specificity of the test has little impact on NPV: all the reported data yield predictive values between 0.92 and 0.97. Similarly, at low prevalence, PPV is low regardless of the sensitivity and specificity data used.

The analysis presented here demonstrates that the MDQ and BSDS perform well at low prevalence (as in the primary care setting), where their strong NPVs can effectively screen out bipolar disorder. When given to a patient who arouses little clinical suspicion of bipolar disorder, a negative MDQ will generally help accomplish just what the US Food and Drug Administration (FDA) has recommended prior to administration of antidepressants: the likelihood of bipolar disorder is low, but will likely be made lower still by the administration of the test.

However, a weakness of these tests is also obvious: a positive result, when the clinician is not very suspicious that bipolar disorder is present, has a very high likelihood of being a false positive. This is so regardless of which sensitivity and specificity data one chooses to use. Yet this is a very likely scenario in primary care if the test is used broadly, e.g. in patients who do not present with depression; or in the bipolar screening the FDA has advocated. Therefore any presentation of the MDQ or BSDS as tools for bipolar screening should be accompanied by a reminder that positive results are not bipolar diagnoses, a point that is sometimes not prominent in pharmaceutical marketing of the MDQ. One available version of the MDQ makes this point to the patient even before the provider scores it.

In sum, the performance of screening instruments such as the MDQ and BSDS depend not only on their sensitivity and specificity, which are properties of the tests themselves, but also on the prevalence of the illness for which one is screening, as predicted by Bayesian principles.

Honing our prior probabilities

I have applied this approach to the problem of difficult diagnoses, such as bipolar disorder in psychiatry. Because prior clinical probability is so important in the process of diagnosing bipolar disorder, it is even more important to acknowledge that clinicians appear to be inadequately trained or proficient in recognizing bipolar disorder. Much more clinical research exists to suggest that bipolar disorder is underdiagnosed than overdiagnosed. The underdiagnosis rate has been confirmed at about 40% in various studies, with about a decade elapsing from the first visit to a mental health professional after an initial manic episode, and the appropriate diagnosis of bipolar disorder. Part of this underdiagnosis likely relates to patients' lack of insight, whereby they deny or fail to describe manic symptoms. Data exist showing that family members report manic symptoms twice as frequently as patients, and thus family report is essential in the diagnostic assessment of bipolar disorder (Goodwin and Jamison, 2007). But in part this is also due to a lack of systematic assessment of hypomanic and manic symptoms on the part of clinicians, in favor of a simpler but fallible "prototype" or "pattern recognition" approach to diagnosis ("she does not look bipolar") (Sprock, 1988). Another common clinical approach which limits diagnostic accuracy is to focus solely on signs or symptoms of mania in assessing the potential diagnosis of bipolar disorder. It is just as important to assess other important diagnostic validators associated with bipolar disorder: family history of bipolar disorder, course of illness (early age of onset, highly recurrent and brief depressive episodes, psychotic depression, postpartum onset), and antidepressant treatment response (especially, mania, tolerance, and non-response) (Goodwin and Jamison, 2007). All of these factors should be considered as a clinician develops his/her "hunch" about the likelihood of bipolarity in a patient. If screening tools are used in lieu of this process, their accuracy will be limited.

It appears from this analysis that a clinician's prior probability estimate (based on clinical history, baseline clinical information, past treatment response, or other clinical impressions) about the likelihood of bipolar disorder in a particular patient has as much impact on the clinical performance of the MDQ or BSDS as the test's sensitivity and specificity (in most cases, more). In practice, clinicians are Bayesians (often without realizing it). If their prior probabilities are low, then these scales more effectively rule out than rule in bipolar disorder. If their prior probabilities are moderate, then these scales may help identify true positive cases. If their prior probabilities are high, then these scales are less relevant. Any improvement in clinicians' ability to form an accurate clinical impression will improve the performance of these tests. Therefore one way to address concerns about the psychometric properties of these screening tests is to help psychiatrists and primary care providers with finding, understanding, and interpreting clinical clues of bipolar disorder.

Bayesian decision-making

John Maynard Keynes is famous as an economist; he arguably saved the world in the Great Depression as he articulated ways that government could ameliorate the capitalist market. Yet, beyond economics, Keynes wrote a major work on probability, and essentially worked out an objectivist approach to Bayesian statistics. Some of his insights in economics may be due to the power of this statistical method.

Clinical medicine would benefit from paying attention to the power of Bayesian statistics. Our current ignorance of it would be as if economists only read Adam Smith and obsessed about the self-regulating aspects of the free market, and never entertained any Keynesian notions about the limitations of the unregulated free market. Bayesian statistics can lead us where frequentist statistics have led us aground. And, perhaps best of all, we clinicians may be more attuned to Bayesian styles of thinking than most statisticians, and thus we can incorporate them more easily.

Put another way, Bayesian statistics provide a way of translating scientific research into practical thinking. For a clinician, a p-value of 0.04 vs. 0.12 tells him very little about how that study should impact his decision-making. Indeed, one of the problems with applying statistics to clinical medicine is that the quantitative power of statistical calculations are often clinically irrelevant. If I say the p-value is 0.038957629376, this highly precise number is no more relevant than p = 0.04. Perhaps even more importantly, clinicians, and human beings in general, cannot make probability discriminations on the order of 5% or 10% or so. We might have the data to make such claims, but the brain of the working clinician cannot "see" such data; the clinician cannot discriminate such data in the real world.

This reality is captured in the large psychological literature on decision-making. Much of this research has to do with concepts such as "heuristics," studies of how people actually make decisions and of how probabilities are actually understood by real people (such as doctors and clinicians) in the real world. One conclusion from this extensive psychological and statistical research on how humans understand probability is that we human beings are able to distinguish only five basic concepts in probability:

> Surely true
> More probable than not
> As probable as not
> Less probable than not
> Surely false

(Salsburg, 2001; p. 307)

Bayesian thinking is a way to get us into these mindsets, to acknowledge how we think, and to help us arrive, as validly as possible, to one of these probability assessments in our clinical practice. Frequentist statistics may want to be more precise, to say that there is a 10%

probability of Y and a 25% probability of Z. But our brains cannot make out that difference. If this is correct, then "many of the techniques of statistical analysis that are standard practice are useless, since they only serve to produce distinctions below the level of human perception." (Salsburg, 2001; p. 307.)

Ultimately, a clinician who wants to understand statistics, and to use it in clinical practice, is ready-made to use Bayesian methods. Bayesian thinking straddles the gulf between the excessive adoration of numbers viewed as truth, so frequent in the world of statistics, and the arbitrary intuitive approach to decision-making for individual patients, the long-held province of the clinician. Instead, Bayesian methods allow clinicians to be more quantitatively sound, and they force statisticians to realize that numbers are not enough. As a Bayesian statistician put it: "Clinical investigators tend to view statisticians as contributing to an investigation by attaching a number to an experiment. Relating the experiment to *medical* questions (how to treat Ms. Smith) is regarded as the purview of medical experts and not of statisticians. A Bayesian approach requires a close working relationship between clinicians and statisticians." (Berry, 1993.) I would go one step further: a Bayesian approach *is* what happens in the work of a statistically informed clinician.

The Bayesian Id

We clinicians are all Bayesians, whether we realize it or not, much as Freud showed that we humans all have unconscious emotions. The statistician Jacob Cohen implied this analogy with his term "the Bayesian Id" (Cohen, 1994).

Here, readers have mulled over the limitations of hypothesis-testing approaches in medical statistics; they have learned about different philosophies of science as they apply to statistics; and they now know what Bayesian statistics mean. After these three steps, readers can perhaps appreciate what Cohen meant when he said that modern statistics has a "hybrid logic," "a mishmash of Fisher and Neyman-Pearson, with invalid Bayesian interpretation." Let me spell this out.

Recall that Fisher invented p-values, and Neyman and Pearson devised the NH method to show how p-values could be used. The two approaches do not necessarily flow: Fisher felt null hypotheses were a conceptual excrescence, and that p-values could stand alone, as long as they were applied in RCTs. We might add that Hill showed, in the debate with Fisher over cigarettes, that RCTs were not sufficient, or even necessary, to prove causation. Modern statistics assumes that p-values and hypothesis-testing are legitimate, but what did Cohen mean by the Bayesian Id?

Perhaps he meant that although we practice the frequentist philosophy of p-values and NH methods, we always, against our will, apply the unconscious Bayesian method of judging the results based on our personal biases. Recall that when we conduct standard frequentist statistics, we ask the question: assuming the NH is true, how likely is it that we would have observed these data? But we tend to interpret the results in reverse: given these observed data, how likely is it that the NH is true? We know we are not supposed to do this; we are told not to do this; but our statistical Id keeps doing it. Cohen makes the point: "When one rejects [the NH], one wants to conclude that [the NH] is unlikely, say, P < .01. The very reason the statistical test is done is to be able to reject [the NH] because of its unlikeliness!" But here we have become Bayesian: we do a study, observe some results, and then try to infer some probability that the NH is false. We are inferring a probability *based on* the data (Bayesian statistics); we are not inferring the probability *of* the data (frequentist statistics): "But that is the posterior probability, available only through Bayes' theorem, for which one needs to know the probability of the null hypothesis before the experiment, the 'prior' probability."

What is the probability of the NH, before we do our study? That is a question never asked by Neyman and Pearson and decades of their disciples in hypothesis-testing statistics. The orthodox answer is: 100%, because we have to *assume* that the NH is correct. But, given that we do research to find new facts, to reject the NH, the reality is that we do not believe that the probability of the NH is 100%. If so, we are forced to engaged in Bayesian reasoning, and we have to provide some prior estimate for the NH, *before* we observe the data.

What could that prior estimate be, without dropping us into the mire of everyone's subjective opinions? As described previously in this chapter, it could be the consensus of previous empirical studies, or the population prevalence of a diagnosis. Whatever it is, we are better off acknowledging the existence of our Bayesian Id, and trying to make it conscious, rather than continuing to live in the dream world of hypothesis-testing statistics.

The unexamined qualitative intuitions that spring from our personal biases are dangerous things. Frequentist statistics wants to imagine as if those subjective parts of research and practice do not exist; Bayesian statistics acknowledges them, and shows us how we can minimize the harm they produce and maximally utilize the availability of objective scientific evidence.

The Reverend Thomas Bayes buried his theorem. Perhaps we should bring it back to life.

The politics of statistics

How journal articles get published

In my journal, anyone can make a fool of himself.

Rudolph Virchow (Silverman, 1998; p. 21)

Perhaps the most important thing to know about scientific publication is that the "best" scientific journals do not publish the most important articles. This will be surprising to some readers, and probably annoying to others (often editorial members of prestigious journals). I could be wrong; this statement reflects my personal experience and my reading of the history of medicine, but if I am correct, the implication for the average clinician is important: it will not be enough to read the largest and most famous journals. For new ideas, one must look elsewhere.

Peer review

The process of publishing scientific articles is a black box to most clinicians and to the public. Unless one engages in research, one would not know all the human foibles that are involved. It is a quite fallible process, but one that seems to have some merit nonetheless.

The key feature is "peer review." The merits of peer review are debatable (Jefferson *et al.*, 2002); indeed its key feature of anonymity can bring out the worst of what has been called the *psychopathology of academe* (Mills, 1963). Let us see how this works.

The process begins when the researcher sends an article to the editor of a scientific journal; the editor then chooses a few (usually 2–4) other researchers who usually are authorities in that topic; those persons are the peer reviewers and they are anonymous. The researcher does not know who they are. These persons then write 1–3 pages of review, detailing specific changes they would like to see in the manuscript. If the paper is not accurate, in their view, or has too many errors, or involves mistaken interpretations, and so on, the reviewers can recommend that it be rejected. The paper would then not be published by that journal, though the researcher could try to send it to a different journal and go through the same process. If the changes requested seem feasible to the editor, then the paper is sent back to the researcher with the specific changes requested by peer reviewers. The researcher can then revise the manuscript and send it back to the editor; if all or most of the changes are made, the paper is then typically accepted for publication. Very rarely, reviewers may recommend acceptance of a paper with no or very minor changes from the beginning.

This is the process. It may seem rational, but the problem is that human beings are involved, and human beings are not, generally, rational. In fact, the whole scientific peer review process is, in my view, quite akin to Winston Churchill's definition of democracy: It is the worst system imaginable, except for all the others.

Perhaps the main problem is what one might call *academic road rage*. As is well known, it is thought that anonymity is a major factor that leads to road rage among drivers of automobiles. When I do not know who the other driver is, I tend to assume the worst about him; and when he cannot see my face, nor I his, I can afford to be socially inappropriate and aggressive, because facial and other physical cues do not impede me. I think the same factors are in play with scientific peer review: routinely, one reads frustrated and angry comments from peer reviewers; exclamation points abound; inferences about one's intentions as an author are made based on pure speculation; one's integrity and research competence are not infrequently questioned. Now sometimes the content that leads to such exasperation is justifiable; legitimate scientific and statistical questions can be raised; it is the emotion and tone which seem excessive.

Four interpretations of peer review

Peer review has become a matter of explicit discussion among medical editors, especially in special issues of the *Journal of the American Medical Association (JAMA)*. The result of this public debate has been summarized as follows:

> Four differing perceptions of the current refereeing process have been identified: 'the sieve (peer review screens worthy from unworthy submissions), the switch (a persistent author can eventually get anything published, but peer review determines where), the smithy (papers are pounded into new and better shapes between the hammer of peer review and the anvil of editorial standards), and the shot in the dark (peer review is essentially unpredictable and unreproducible and hence, in effect, random).' It is remarkable that there is little more than opinion to support these characterizations of the gate-keeping process which plays such a critical role in the operation of today's huge medical research enterprise ('peer review is the linch pin of science.').
>
> (Silverman, 1998; p. 27)

I tend to subscribe to the "switch" and "smithy" interpretations. I do not think that peer review is the wonderful sieve of the worthy from the unworthy that so many assume, nor is it simply random.

It is humanly irrational, however, and thus a troublesome "linchpin" for our science.

It is these human weaknesses that trouble me. For instance, peer reviewers often know authors, either personally or professionally, and they may have a personal dislike for an author; or if not, they may dislike the author's ideas, in a visceral and emotional way. (For all we know, some may also have economic motivations, as some critics of the pharmaceutical industry suggest [Healy, 2001].) How can we remove these biases inherent in anonymous peer review? One approach would be to remove anonymity, and force peer reviewers to identify themselves. Since all authors are peer reviewers for others, and all peer reviewers also write their own papers as authors, editors would be worried that they would not get complete and direct critiques from peer reviewers, who might fear retribution by authors (when serving as peer reviewers). Not just paper publication, but grant funding – money, the life blood of a person's employment in medical research – are subject to anonymous peer review, and thus grudges that might be expressed in later peer review could in fact lead to losing funding and consequent economic hardship.

Who reviews the reviewers?

We see how far we have come from the neutral objective ideals of science. The scientific peer review process involves human beings of flesh and blood, who like and dislike each other, and the dollar bill, here as elsewhere, has a pre-eminent role.

How good or bad is this anonymous peer review process? I have described the matter qualitatively; are there any statistical studies of it? There are, in fact; one study for example, decided to "review the reviewers" (Baxt *et al.*, 1998). All reviewers of the *Annals of Emergency Medicine* received a fictitious manuscript, a purported placebo-controlled randomized clinical trial of a treatment for migraine, in which 10 major and 13 minor statistical and scientific errors were deliberately placed. (Major errors included no definition of migraine, absence of any inclusion or exclusion criteria, and use of a rating scale that had never been validated or previously reported. Also, the p-values reported for the main outcome were made up and did not follow in any way from the actual data presented. The data demonstrated no difference between drug and placebo, but the authors concluded that there was a difference.) Of about 200 reviewers, 15 recommended acceptance of the manuscript, 117 rejection, and 67 revision. So about half of reviewers appropriately realized that the manuscript had numerous flaws, beyond the amount that would usually allow for appropriate revision. Further, 68% of reviewers did not realize that the conclusions written by the manuscript authors did not follow from other results of the study.

If this is the status of scientific peer review, then one has to be concerned that many studies are poorly vetted, and that some of the published literature (at least) is inaccurate either in its exposition or its interpretation.

Mediocrity rewarded

Beyond the publication of papers that should not be published, the peer review process has the problem of not publishing papers that should be published. In my experience both as an author and as an occasional guest editor for scientific journals, when multiple peer reviews bring up different concerns, it is impossible for authors to respond adequately to a wide range of critiques, and thus difficult for editors to publish. In such cases, the problem, perhaps, is not so much the content of the paper, but rather the topic itself. It may be too controversial, or too new, and thus difficult for several peer reviewers to agree that it merits publication.

In my own writing, I have noticed that, at times, the most rejected papers are the most enduring. My rule of thumb is that if a paper is rejected more than five times, then it is either completely useless or utterly prescient. In my view, scientific peer review ousts poor papers – but also great ones; the middling, comfortably predictable, tend to get published.

This brings us back to the claim at the beginning of this chapter, that the most prestigious journals usually do not publish the most original or novel articles; this is because the peer review process is inherently conservative. I do not claim that there is any better system, but I think the weaknesses of our current system need to be honestly acknowledged.

One weakness is that scientific innovation is rarely welcomed, and new ideas are always at a disadvantage against the old and staid. Again, non-researchers might have had a more favorable illusion about science, that it encourages progress and new ideas and that it is consciously self-critical. That is how it should be; but this is how it is, again in the words of Ronald Fisher:

> A scientific career is peculiar in some ways. Its raison d'être is the increase of natural knowledge. Occasionally, therefore, an increase of natural knowledge occurs. But this is tactless, and feelings are hurt. For in some small degree it is inevitable that views previously expounded are shown to be either obsolete or false. Most people, I think, can recognize this and take it in good part if what they have been teaching for ten years or so comes to need a little revision; but some undoubtedly take it hard, as a

blow to their *amour propre*, or even as an invasion of the territory they have come to think of as exclusively their own, and they must react with the same ferocity as we can see in the robins and chaffinches these spring days when they resent an intrusion into their little territories. I do not think anything can be done about it. It is inherent in the nature of our profession; but a young scientist may be warned and advised that when he has a jewel to offer for the enrichment of mankind some certainly will wish to turn and rend him.

(Salsburg, 2001; p. 51)

So this is part of the politics of science – how papers get published. It is another aspect of statistics where we see numbers give way to human emotions, where scientific law is replaced by human arbitrariness. Even with all these limitations, we somehow manage to see a scientific literature that produces useful knowledge. The wise clinician will use that knowledge where possible, while aware of the limitations of the process.

Chapter 16

How scientific research impacts practice

A drug is a substance that, when injected into a rat, produces a scientific paper.
Edgerton Y. Davis (Mackay, 1991; p. 69)

The almighty impact factor

Many practitioners may not know that there is a private company, Thomson Reuters, owner of ISI (Information Sciences Institute), which calculates in a rather secretive fashion a quantitative score that drives much scientific research. This score, called the impact factor (IF), reflects how frequently papers are cited in the references of other papers. The more frequently papers are cited, presumably the more "impact" they are having on the world of research and practice. This calculation is relevant both for journals and for researchers. For journals, the more its articles are cited, the higher its IF, the greater its prestige, which, as with all things in our wonderfully capitalist world, translates into money: advertisers and subscribers flock to the journals with the highest prestige, the greatest … impact. I participate in scientific journal editorial boards, and I have heard editors describe quite explicitly and calmly how they want to elicit more and more papers that are likely to have a high IF. Thus, given two papers that might be equally valid and solid scientifically, with one being on a "sexy" topic that generates much public interest, and another on a "non-sexy" topic, all other things being equal, the editor will lean towards the article that will interest readers more. Now this is not in itself open to criticism: we expect editors of popular magazines and newspapers to do the same; my point is that many clinicians and the public see science as such a stuffy affair that they may not realize that similar calculations go into the scientific publication process.

The IF also matters to individual researchers. Just as baseball players have batting averages by which their skills are judged, the IF is, in a way, a statistical batting average for medical researchers. In fact, ISI ranks researchers and produces a top ten list of the most cited scientific authors in each discipline. In psychiatry, for instance, the most cited author tends to be the first author of large epidemiological studies. Why is he cited so frequently? Because every time one writes a scientific article about depression, and begins with a generic statement such as "Major depressive disorder is a common condition, afflicting 10% of the US population," that first author of the main epidemiological studies of mental illness frequency is likely to be cited. Does such research move mountains? Not really. There is, no doubt, some relevance to the IF and some correlation with the value of scientific articles. There are data to back up this notion. Apparently, about 50% of scientific articles are never cited even once. The median rate of citation is only 1–2 citations. Fifty to one hundred citations would put an article above the 99th percentile, and over 100 citations is the hallmark of a "classic" paper (Carroll, 2006).

So IF captures something, but its correlation with quality research is not as strong or as direct as one might assume. One analysis looked at 131 articles publishing randomized clinical trials (RCTs), and found that the quality of the studies was the same regardless of the IF (Barbui *et al.*, 2006). Poorly cited studies were just as scientifically rigorous as highly cited ones.

So IF must involve something more than research quality: this is where the politics of science is relevant. Topics that are in the public eye will have greater IFs; researchers who are already well-established, and thus known to colleagues through conferences and personal contact, may have their work cited more frequently than unknown authors; and large research groups may inflate the IF scores of their colleagues by citing each other liberally in their publications. The rich get richer.

The distorting effect of the impact factor

One of my friends, currently a chairman of a department of psychiatry, described how his previous chair would sit down at "Google Scholar" and put in his name, and that of my friend, and whoever else was standing around, so as to compare the number of citations of the most popular papers each had published. In this way, scientific prestige, which used to be a more intuitively established matter, has become quantified. But the frequency with which people say one's name does not necessarily entail that one has much of importance to say.

The potential "distorting influence" of the IF on scientific research has begun to be recognized (Brown, 2007). The decline in clinical research in medicine is especially relevant: clinical research is much less funded than basic animal research, and there are far fewer faculty members in medical schools who are clinical researchers, as opposed to basic science researchers. Some think that this process is hastened because papers published by basic science researchers are more frequently cited by other scientists (and thus have a higher IF) than papers published by clinical researchers (Brown, 2007). By judging faculty for promotion and retention based on the "impact" of their publications, medical schools would thus overestimate basic researchers and conversely underestimate the impact of clinical researchers. The IF is an imperfect and gross measure of the value of research, but "everyone loves a number" (Brown, 2007).

The intangibles of co-authorship

Another aspect of the politics of science is self-censorship on the part of co-authors. Especially with large research papers (and perhaps more so if they are co-written by employees or hires of the pharmaceutical industry), the interpretation of results tends to be driven in the favorable direction. This may be for various reasons: an obvious one is pecuniary interests when a study is pharmaceutically funded, but other more intangible reasons may be just as important. Especially for large RCTs, much money has been spent by someone (whether by taxpayers or pharmaceutical executives), and authors may feel a need to justify that expense. Further, such RCTs often take years to complete, and there are only so many years in a person's life; thus authors may feel a need to think that they have been spending their lives wisely, producing important scientific results rather than failed data or debatable findings. The first authors tend to have spent more effort in such large studies than later authors, and thus they tend to drive the interpretive forces of published papers. In an interesting qualitative study (Horton, 2002a), a researcher found that 67% of contributors to research articles expressed reservations and concerns to him which they had not presented in the published paper. A certain amount of self-censorship seemed to be happening.

The published peer review process: letters to the editor

One might expect the anonymous peer review process to bring out such limitations before papers are published, but as described in Chapter 15 the peer review process can, and not infrequently does, fail in some measure. A secondary back-up is the process of reaction in published letters to the editor after the publication of a scientific paper. One limitation here is that such letters are no longer anonymous, and thus the potential for personal animosity is raised, probably leading to a certain amount of withholding of public criticism by other researchers. Nonetheless, even with this limitation, one would expect that published letters to the editor, and responses to them by researchers, would further allow the published scientific literature to be better analyzed and weaknesses and flaws better known. One problem with this aspect of science, though, is that letters to the editor are not abstracted in computerized search engines (such as Medline) and they are not available in computerized format (such as .pdf files) via the internet. Thus, readers interested in a certain study after the fact would have to go old-school, trudging to the library to find hard copies of journals, if they actually wished to read the letters to the editor reacting to a published study. These days, such efforts are undertaken less and less in the busy world of internet-driven scientific research. Even if someone bothered to read the published letters and investigator responses, one study finds that more than half of the specific criticisms found in letters to the editor are left unanswered by the authors of published studies (Horton, 2002b). That analysis found that when compared to the impact of important published studies on later treatment guidelines, critiques presented in letters to the editor rarely are acknowledged or incorporated in clinical practice guidelines.

In sum, the scientific publication process involves human judgment, subjectivity, and interpretation – just like statistics. Numbers do not capture the whole thing.

Chapter 17

Dollars, data, and drugs

There's an old saying that victory has a hundred fathers and defeat is an orphan.
John F. Kennedy (Kennedy, 1962)

What should we believe?

One cannot honestly write about statistics these days, without confronting the pachyderm in the room. Much has been made in recent years about the baneful influence of the pharmaceutical industry on medical research, and statistics, as enshrined in the evidence-based medicine (EBM) movement (some call it "evidence-biased medicine"), is seen as an accomplice.

It is not new for statistics to be viewed with suspicion, as described previously, long before the first pharmaceutical company ever existed. Indeed, it has long been known that statistics are prone to being misused; witness the famous comment by the nineteenth-century British prime minister Disraeli about lies, damn lies, and statistics.

This amenability to abuse is inherent in the nature of statistics; it can happen because using statistics is not just about the dry application of clear-cut rules, as many clinicians seem to assume. By now, in this book, this fact should be clear: statistics are chock full of assumptions and concepts and interpretations. In a word, numbers do not stand by themselves.

I am perennially surprised by the shock expressed by clinicians when they find that the pharmaceutical industry has messed around with statistics and science, as if the process of science somehow went on in an ether above our base world of humans and passions and economics and faiths. There should be no shock, but there also should be no wholesale rejection, thereby, of statistics and science. I hear clinicians repeatedly say: "I don't know who to believe anymore; so I won't believe anything." But it is not a matter of *belief*: it is a matter of science, properly conceived. It is not enough to say that we cannot believe scientific studies at face value, and then to reject them all; we must learn how to *evaluate* them so that we know which ones to believe and which ones to discount.

That is a major reason why I wrote this book. I believe the answer to the harmful influence of the pharmaceutical industry in medical research is to become less ignorant about medical research. If we as clinicians knew more, we would not be so open to being manipulated.

I expect, however, that critics of the pharmaceutical industry and cynics about statistics would view this book as incomplete unless I acknowledged and addressed the various ways in which that branch of free market capitalism affects the research enterprise – a not unreasonable request.

Ghost authorship

The first specter that we need to acknowledge is ghost authorship. This is the process whereby pharmaceutical companies draft scientific papers, later published under the "authorship" of academic researchers. I have seen this process from the inside. Usually, it occurs in the setting of a pharmaceutically designed multi-center clinical trial. The pharmaceutical company actually designs and writes the study protocol, often meant for US Food and Drug Administration (FDA) registration for a new drug. The company then recruits a number of academic and research sites to help conduct the study, get the patients who will enter it, and give the treatments and collect outcomes. The data that are produced are collected in a central site in the pharmaceutical company, analyzed by employee statisticians there. If the study shows no benefit, the process usually ends here. The results are never published (unpublished negative studies are discussed below), the drug is not taken to the FDA since it will be rejected, and the company turns to studying other drugs. If the results show that the drug is effective, then the company takes the data to the FDA for an official "indication" so that it can be marketed to the public. To publish the data in a scientific journal, the company often hires a medical writing company to prepare a first draft manuscript based on the data analysis by its statisticians. Then researchers who were part of the study, those who had recruited patients for it and led its various research sites, are asked to be co-authors on the paper, and often they receive payments to be co-authors. They read the first draft manuscript, make suggestions for revision, and the company writers revise the paper accordingly. When submitted for publication in a scientific journal, the resulting paper does not usually have the name of any company employees or any individuals in the medical writing company. (Sometimes, in the middle or towards the end of the co-author list, the company statistician and/or physician employees of the pharmaceutical company will be listed.) Usually, the first author and the following top authors are the most senior and recognized academic leaders among those who had participated in designing and executing the study. Their role is often seen as legitimizing the study and lending the weight of their authority, as "key opinion leaders" (Moynihan, 2008), to the results.

In the best conditions, I have observed, as a middle author among a list of ten or more co-authors, that usually most comments for revision come from the first or second author, and rarely from most of the other co-authors. And if the majority of authors make comments, they are usually quite minor. In effect, most co-authors are silent accomplices on the published paper. For them, it has the advantage of padding their resumés with one more paper, usually highly cited and published in prestigious journals (Patsopoulos *et al.*, 2006). These resumés more quickly will appear to merit academic promotion to senior professorship positions. Critics of the pharmaceutical industry see, rightly in my view, an unholy alliance where both sides benefit, at the cost of truth.

In worse circumstances, matters are even more concerning. I will relate two of my personal experiences.

Personal experience

Once, a pharmaceutical company asked me to be first author of a paper derived from a large randomized clinical trial (RCT) in bipolar disorder. (Often one RCT leads to multiple publications, as the company tries to highlight different secondary outcomes in each succeeding publication.) I agreed, and received a completed first draft of the manuscript, in which a secondary outcome of cognition was reported to be improved by the drug. I noted that the patients' mood had also improved with drug, so it was not clear whether the improved cognition was a direct effect of the drug, or an indirect effect of improving mood. I asked for more statistical analysis using regression modeling to control for the improvement in mood. My hypothesis was that cognition improved due to improvement in mood, and that the drug was otherwise neutral in its direct effect on mood. My counterpart in the company told me that there was not enough time to continue analyzing the paper extensively; the company had a timeline for publication, and since the peer review process can be slow, they needed to move forward to journal submission. I removed myself as first author, and about 6 months later the paper was published, largely unchanged, with another person as first author.

On another occasion, a colleague asked me to be second author on an RCT for a study with which I had never had any relationship, either initially in designing the protocol or later as a study site during its execution. They just wanted to add my name among the co-authors. I declined.

A few years later, during an academic review, the psychiatry department leadership where I worked noted that I did not have many publications that were RCTs, which they felt weakened my scholarly standing for future promotion. I was left unpleasantly aware that these rejected publications, handed to me on a platter, were the kinds of citations that these leaders had used to reach their positions.

Who has the data?

One other factor is important: as described above, in almost all cases of large RCTs, the authors do not themselves analyze the data statistically; the analyses are conducted by company statisticians. When I have asked for access to the data myself, I am told that they are proprietary: private property, in effect, upon which I cannot trespass. Thus, unless the FDA requests them, scientists and the public can never confirm the actual data analyses themselves. One need not imagine actual data tampering, which would obviously be illegal, but, given our knowledge that statistics involve subjectivity, one can imagine analyses that are done and not reported, and analyses that are not reported exactly as they were done. For instance, an RCT may report a post-hoc positive result with a p-value of 0.01, but we have no denominator. We do not know if it was one positive result out of 5, or 335, analyses.

Proof of ghost authorship

Beyond personal experience, it is hard to prove or quantify the extent and effects of ghost authorship, because much of what happens occurs behinds the proprietary walls of the private sector, in contrast to the public workings of academic science. The only means of getting behind those walls are governmental or legal injunctions. Such access recently occurred with legal processes in relation to the anti-inflammatory drug rofecoxib (Vioxx) (Ross et al., 2008). Reviewing 250 internal documents, researchers were able to show how the process unfolds as I have described above. Further, although companies would acknowledge sponsoring studies, researchers found that only 50% (36 of 72) of relevant ghost-written articles disclosed company involvement in authorship or that the published authors had received honoraria. If this result were to be generalized to the entire scientific literature, approximately one-half of

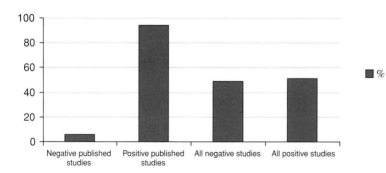

Figure 17.1 FDA database of antidepressant RCTs for unipolar depression: comparison of studies published from that database and all studies in the database (including unpublished studies).

all pharmaceutically sponsored articles are ghost-written. Other evidence suggests that about one-third of the clinical research literature is pharmaceutically sponsored (Buchkowsky and Jewesson, 2004). Thus, one might estimate that about 20% of the clinical research literature is ghost-written. If true, this raises concerns that some medical science is "McScience" (Horton, 2004), a junk version of the real thing. Major journals are well aware of these problems (Davidoff *et al.*, 2001), but so far academic medicine has not made a coordinated effort to end ghost authorship.

Unpublished negative studies

It is now well demonstrated that pharmaceutical industry sponsorship of studies correlates with positive results for the agent being studied (Lexchin *et al.*, 2003). Some clinicians may mistakenly see this as the result of cheating: the data must be rigged. In fact, it reflects something more subtle, producing the same result: suppression of negative studies.

Clinical example 1: antidepressant RCTs

This process has been best documented in a recent review of the FDA database of all 74 antidepressant clinical trials for unipolar depression in over 12 000 subjects. Forty-nine percent of studies were negative, and 51% were positive (Turner *et al.*, 2008). Yet since most negative studies were unpublished, the published literature was 94% positive (see Figure 17.1).

Further, of the negative studies, 61% were unpublished, 8% were published as frankly negative, but 31% were published as positive! This is usually where the negative primary outcomes are underplayed or even ignored, where the distinction between primary and secondary outcomes is not admitted, and where positive secondary outcomes are presented as if they were the main result of the study.

Unless a drug eventually receives FDA indication, a company is not required to provide all its data on that drug, including negative studies, to the FDA or anyone else. Thus, many drugs are simply ineffective, and proven so, but if they do not have an FDA indication for that condition, no one will know.

It is worth noting that a few exceptions exist, where academic authors have published negative studies on a drug, but usually multiple negative RCTs are combined in one published paper (Pande *et al.*, 2000; Kushner *et al.*, 2006), producing much less impact than the usual multiple publications that ensue out of a positive single RCT (with positive results usually found in the most read, most prestigious journals).

Clinical example 2: lamotrigine in bipolar disorder

The pharmaceutical industry has not yet made its negative data available routinely and fully on its websites, and where such data are available, again as the result of litigation, important evidence of clinical inefficacy can be found (Ghaemi *et al.*, 2008a). For instance, among the major companies with agents indicated for bipolar disorder, only GlaxoSmithKline (GSK) has provided data on its website regarding unpublished negative studies with results that were unfavorable to their product lamotrigine (Lamictal). Of nine studies provided at the GSK website, two were positive and published, and supported the company's success in securing an FDA-approved indication for lamotrigine for delay of relapse in the long-term treatment of bipolar disorder patients (Bowden *et al.*, 2003; Calabrese *et al.*, 2003). Two negative studies have been published, one in rapid-cycling (Calabrese *et al.*, 2000) and another in acute bipolar depression (Calabrese *et al.*, 1999), but both published versions emphasize positive secondary outcomes as opposed to the negative primary outcomes. A negative study in rapid-cycling has not been published in detail (GW611), nor have two negative randomized studies in acute bipolar depression (GW40910 and GW603), as well as two negative randomized trials in acute mania (GW609 and GW610). A recent meta-analysis of five negative studies in acute bipolar depression is another example of the alchemy of turning dross to gold: when the five samples of about 200 patients each are pooled, the total sample of about 1000 patients produces a positive p-value – but, not surprisingly, with a tiny effect size (about one point improvement on the Hamilton Depression Rating Scale) (Calabrese *et al.*, 2008).

The clinical relevance of the lamotrigine studies is notable: taking the negative outcomes into account, as of now, one might say that this agent is quite effective in maintenance treatment of bipolar disorder, but it is not effective in acute mania, or rapid-cycling, or perhaps acute bipolar depression. This context of where the drug is effective, and where it is not, is vital for scientifically valid and ethically honest clinical practice and research.

Disease-mongering

Another aspect of clinical research that has come under scrutiny is the creation and expansion of diagnostic categories. Some critics argue that instead of discovering drugs for our diseases, we are creating diseases to match our drugs (Moynihan *et al.*, 2002). This propensity seems most likely with single symptom diagnoses, such as ADHD or social anxiety disorder. It has been claimed that even traditional diagnoses of centuries standing, such as bipolar disorder, may also be prone to it (Healy, 2008). Although disease-mongering happens, many critics are so perturbed that they appear to suffer from the *disease of seeing disease-mongering everywhere*, and argue that any increase in diagnosis of anything represents disease-mongering. Some diseases have been and are underdiagnosed: bipolar disorder is one of them, AIDS is another. Increases in diagnoses of those conditions may reflect improved diagnostic practice.

Nonetheless, sometimes the marketing influence of pharmaceutically oriented research may not be directly about treatment studies, but rather about studies which promote increased diagnosis relevant to the treatment in question. Some have blamed the EBM movement for these practices, even though most EBM concepts are not related to diagnostic studies. While I have not addressed specifics of diagnostic research in this book, it is relevant that some of these questionable marketing-oriented research practices can be critiqued by using Bayesian concepts, as I did in analysis of studies of the Mood Disorder Questionnaire in Chapter 14.

Follow the money

Some critics have appeared to become proto-Marxists, insisting that the only factor that matters is economics. Follow the money, they say (Abramson, 2004). If a doctor has any relationship with any pharmaceutical company funding, he must be biased; one author even advises patients to fire their doctors on this ground alone (Angell, 2005). This kind of postmodernist criticism – seeing nothing but power and money as the source of all knowledge – seems simplistic, to say the least (Dennett, 2000). Even government funding can be related to bias. It may be in fact that the bias has less to do with funding than with researchers' own belief-systems, their ideologies (another concept derivable from Karl Marx). This is a complex topic, but a source of evidence that argues against an economic reductionist model is that about one-quarter of all psychiatric research is not even funded at all, *by any source* (Silberman and Snyderman, 1997). Often those unfunded studies are sources of important new ideas.

Avoiding nihilism

These critiques are not meant to engender a nihilistic reaction in the reader. It is not necessary to think nothing is meaningful simply because science is complex. Having read this far, readers should not conclude that the scientific literature is useless. They should, I hope, use this book to be able to navigate the scientific literature. There are more than enough voices on the internet and elsewhere of those who take a one-sided view: everything is horrible; or everything is perfect. The truth is never so simple.

Thinking back to the first section of this book, where I highlighted that all facts are theory-laden, it may also be relevant to point out that the influence of bias in clinical research is not limited to the pharmaceutical industry. Even government-funded studies can be biased for the simple reason that, although money is influential human beings are also motivated by other desires: chief among these is prestige, which from Plato to Hegel has been recognized as perhaps the ultimate human desire. Many researchers, subtly or obviously, consciously or unconsciously, are biased by their wish to be right. Sometimes the truth takes a backseat when defending one's opinions. It is quite difficult for any person to be fully free of this hubris. Sometimes, it completely takes over and destroys one. A sobering example, useful to show how influences other than money can matter, is a prominent case of a PhD researcher who specialized in diabetes research. For a decade he obtained numerous National Institute of Health (NIH) grants which led to much prestige; his research was not unusual; in fact he apparently doctored his data so that his results would agree with the academic mainstream, thus ensuring him more governmental funding and academic prestige (Sox and Rennie, 2006). He went to prison.

Researcher bias can, and does, occur for many reasons. While efforts are needed to clean up academic medicine, clinicians will always need to hone and use their ultimate tool: knowledge.

Chapter 18

Bioethics and the clinician/researcher divide

> Almost everyone can and should do research ... because almost everyone has a unique observational opportunity at some time in his life which he has an obligation to record ... If one considers the fundamental operations or methods of research, one immediately realizes that most people do research at some time or another, except that they do not call their activity by that name.
>
> John Cade (Cade, 1971)

An underlying theme of this book is that one cannot be a good clinician unless one understands research. I also believe the opposite holds for clinical research: one cannot be a good clinical researcher unless one is an active clinician.

The divide that exists between the world of clinical practice and the world of research is partly the result of lack of knowledge; the main purpose of this book is to redress that lack of knowledge on the part of clinicians. But partly also the divide is widened due to biases and, in my view, a mistaken approach, by the mainstream bioethics community, to the ethics of research.

The biases of some non-researchers toward clinical research became clear to me in one of my academic positions. A leader in our department was a prominent psychoanalyst, an active clinician who had never conducted research. He was convinced that *any* research activity must, by that mere fact, be ethically suspect. This is because clinical work is done in the interests of the patient, while research is done in the interests of knowledge (society, science; not the individual patient). This is the basic belief of mainstream bioethics, enforced daily by the institutional review boards of all academic centers, and policed by the federal government.

Yet if John Cade was right, then something is awry, and the problem of clinical innovation highlights the matter.

Clinical innovation

Most clinicians, researchers, and ethicists would agree that it is important to expand medical knowledge, and thus, at a very basic level, it is ethical to engage in research, given appropriate protections for research subjects. As a corollary, one might argue that it is unethical *not* to do research. We must, as a result, constantly be aware of the need to balance the risk of being ignorant versus the risks involved in obtaining new knowledge. Too often, this debate is one-sided, focused on the risks involved in obtaining new knowledge. But there are risks on both sides of the ledger, and not doing research poses real risks also. Hence the importance of assessing the merits of clinical innovation, which I believe is a legitimate component of the research process.

Virtually everything that gets to clinical trials comes from early clinical innovation. Conceived in terms used by evidence-based medicine (EBM), innovation in psychopharmacology more commonly proceeds bottom-up, rather than top-down (Table 3.1). Innovation proceeds usually from level V case reports, through levels III–IV naturalistic and non-randomized studies, to levels I–II randomized studies.

Clinical innovation occurs, by definition, outside of formal research protocols. There is a risk that guidelines of any kind, however well-intentioned, will impede clinical innovation unnecessarily. On the other hand, there are limits to acceptable innovation, and in some cases, one can imagine cases of innovation that would appear to be unethical.

The Belmont Report

Part of the problem is that the bioethics community has sought to cleanly and completely separate clinical practice from research. In the *Belmont Report of The National Commission for the Protection of Human Subjects* (National Institute of Health, 1979), for instance, an attempt was made to separate "practice," where "interventions are designed solely to enhance the wellbeing of an individual patient or client and that have a reasonable expectation of success," from "research," defined as "an activity designed to test an hypothesis, permit conclusions to be drawn, and thereby to develop or contribute to generalizable knowledge." In fact, the clinician/researcher engaging in clinical innovation is not acting with solely one set of interests in mind, but two. On the one hand, the clinician/researcher wants to help the individual patient; on the other hand, the clinician/researcher wants to gain some experience or knowledge from his/her observation. Some in the bioethics community set up this scenario as a necessary conflict. They seem to think that a choice must be made: either the clinician must choose to seek only to make the patient better, without learning anything in the process, or the clinician must seek to learn something, without any intention at all to improve the patient's lot. As with so much in life, there are in fact multiple interests here and there is no need to insist that those interests do not overlap at all. First and foremost in any clinical encounter is the clinician's responsibility to the individual welfare of the patient. Any innovative treatment, observation, or hypothesis cannot be allowed to lead to complete lack of regard for the patient's welfare. Unfortunately, the Belmont Report and much of the mainstream bioethics literature presumes complete and unavoidable conflict of these interests: "When a clinician departs in a significant way from standard or accepted practice, the innnovation does not, in and of itself, constitute research. The fact that a procedure is 'experimental', in the sense of new, untested, or different, does not automatically place it in the category of research ... [but] the general rule is that if there is any element of research in an activity, that activity should undergo review for the protection of human subjects."

This approach leads, in my view, to uncontrolled clinical innovation and overregulated formal research. The ultimate rationale for clinical innovation lies in the history of the many serendipitous discoveries of medical practice. Psychopharmacology is full of such stories, Cade's discovery of lithium being perhaps the paradigm case.

Cade's discovery of lithium

In the 1940s, John Cade hypothesized that mania and depression represented abnormalities of nitrogen metabolism. He injected urine samples from psychiatric patients into guinea pigs, all of whom died. He concluded that the nitrogenous product, urea, was probably acting as a poison, and later tested uric acid solubilized as lithium urate, which led to marked calming of the guinea pigs. Further tests identified lithium to be the calming agent, and Cade then proceeded to try lithium himself before giving it to patients. His first patient improved markedly, but then experienced toxicity and died after a year. Cade was quite concerned and abandoned using lithium further due to its toxicity, but reported his findings in detail. Other researchers, in the first randomized clinical trials (RCTs) in psychiatry, proved lithium safe and effective at non-toxic levels.

Would we have lithium if Cade were working today? It is unlikely.

It is striking that there is a double standard here: attempts to expand knowledge that are labeled "research" receive intense scrutiny, whereas clinical innovation receives no scrutiny at all. One researcher commented that if he wanted to give a new drug to half of his patients (in an RCT), he would need to go through miles of administrative ethical hoops, but if he wanted to give a new drug to all of his patients, nothing stood in his way. Something is wrong with this scenario.

Trivial research, thoughtless practice

At the National Institute of Mental Health (NIMH), research funding has been divided between "intramural" and "extramural" types. Extramural research required extensive oversight into scientific utility. Intramural research did not require such oversight and was designed to encourage innovative ideas. In the terminology of Steve Brodie, an icon of Nobel-prize level psychiatric research, intramural research allowed investigators to "take a flier" on new ideas (Kanigel, 1986). Unfortunately, now intramural research at the NIMH requires extramural-like levels of scientific oversight and justification. As a result, both inside the NIMH and outside psychiatric research is more and more comprised of *increasing pristine presentations of increasingly trivial points* (Ghaemi and Goodwin, 2007).

The NIMH has also tended to avoid funding of clinical psychopharmacology research on the grounds that a source of funds exists in private industry; the limitations of that attitude are now well known (see Chapter 17).

Some will argue that my discussion of clinical innovation here conflicts with federal standards, such as the *Belmont Report*, which has been identified by the National Institutes of Health (NIH) Office of Human Subjects Research as the philosophical foundation for its ethical regulations (Forster, 1979). After all, we have to follow the law.

As mentioned above, the Report leaves itself open to a strict interpretation when it asserts that "any element of research" requires formal review. However, the Report also establishes three fundamental ethical principles that are relevant to all research involving human subjects: respect for persons, beneficence, and justice. One could argue that the status quo, by overregulating research and ignoring clinical practice, is not in keeping with the principles underlying the Belmont Report. Even the NIH notes that the Report is "not a set of rules that can be applied rigidly to make determinations of whether a proposed research activity is ethically 'right' or 'wrong.' Rather, these regulations provide a framework in which investigators and others can ensure that serious efforts have been made to protect the rights and welfare of research subjects."

I think the best research is conducted by active clinicians, and that the best clinical work is conducted by active researchers. The strict wall separating pure research from pure clinical practice is at best a fiction, and at worst a dumbing down of both activities. A change in some of the basic axioms of the field of research ethics may be needed so that we can avoid the alternative extremes of indiscriminate clinical practice on the one hand and overregulation of all research on the other.

A coda by A. Bradford Hill

It may be fitting to end this book by letting A. Bradford Hill again speak to us, now on this topic of so great concern to him: bringing clinicians and researchers together, combining medicine and statistics. He saw room for both statisticians and clinicians to learn to come together (Hill, 1962; pp. 31–2):

> In my indictment of the statistician, I would argue that he may tend to be a trifle too scornful of the clinical judgment, the clinical impression. Such judgments are, I believe, in essence, statistical. The clinician is attempting to make a comparison between the situation that faces him at the moment and a mentally recorded but otherwise untabulated past experience … Turning now to the other side of the picture – the attitude of the clinician – I would, from experience, say that the most frequent and the most foolish criticism of the statistical approach in medicine is that human beings are too variable to allow of the contrasts inherent in a controlled trial of a remedy. In other words, each patient is 'unique' and so there can be nothing for the statistician to count. But if this is true it has always seemed to me that the bottom falls out of the clinical approach as well as the statistical. If each patient is unique, how can a basis for treatment be found in the past observations of other patients?

Hill goes on to note that each patient is not totally unique from another patient, but many variable features differ among patients. This produces, through confounding bias, the messy result of unscientific medicine, full of competing opinions and observations:

> Two or three uncontrolled observations may, therefore, give merely through the customary play of chance, a favourable picture in the hands of one doctor, an unfavourable picture in the hands of a second. And so the medical journals, euphemistically called the 'literature', are cluttered up with conflicting claims – each in itself perfectly true of what the doctor saw, and each insufficient to bear the weight of the generalization placed upon it. Far, therefore, from arguing that the statistical approach is impossible in the face of human variability, we should realize that it is because of that variability that it is often essential.

The sum of it all is this: one cannot be a good clinician unless one is a good researcher, and one cannot be a good researcher unless one is a good clinician. Good clinical practice shares all the features of good research: careful observation, attention to bias and chance, replication, reasoned inference of causation.

We are still in limbo, "until that happy day arrives when every clinician is his own statistician," as Hill put it (Hill, 1962; p. 30), but we will never reach that day until we become aware that medicine without statistics is quackery, and statistics without medicine is numerology.

Appendix: Regression models and multivariable analysis

Assumptions of regression models

The use of regression models involves some layers of complexity beyond those discussed in the text. To recapitulate: "Multivariable analysis is a statistical tool for determining the unique contributions of various factors to a single event or outcome." (Katz, 2003.) Its rationale is that one cannot answer all questions with randomized studies: "In many clinical situations, experimental manipulation of study groups would be unfeasible, unethical, or impractical...For example, we cannot test whether smoking increases the likelihood of coronary artery disease by randomly assigning persons to groups who smoke and do not smoke." (Katz, 2003.)

The rationale and benefits of multivariable regression are clear, but it too has limitations. There are three types of regression: linear (for continuous outcomes, such as change in depression rating scale score), logistic (for dichotomous outcomes, such as being a responder or not), and Cox (for time to event outcomes, as in survival analysis).

In *linear* regression, there is an assumption "that, as the independent variables increase (or decrease), the mean value of the outcome increases (or decreases) in linear fashion." (Katz, 2003.) Non-linear relationships would not be accurately captured in a regression model; sometimes statisticians will "transform" the variables with logarithmic or other changes to the regression equation, so as to convert a non-linear relationship between the outcome and the predictors to a linear relationship. This is not inherently problematic, but it is complex and it involves changing the data more and more from their original presentation. Sometimes these transformations still fail to create a linear relationship, and in such cases, the non-linear reality cannot be captured with standard linear regression models.

In *logistic* regression, "the basic assumption is that each one-unit increase in a predictor multiplies the odds of the outcome by a certain factor (the odds ratio of the predictor) and that the effect of several variables is the multiplicative product of their individual effects." (Katz, 2003.) If the combined effect of several variables is additive or exponential, rather than simply multiplicative, the logistic regression model will not accurately capture that relationship of those several variables to the outcome.

In *Cox* regression, there is a proportionality assumption: "the ratio of the hazard functions for persons with and without a given risk factor is the same over the entire study period." (Katz, 2003.) This means that two groups – say one who receives antidepressants and one who does not – would differ in a constant amount in risk of relapse over a period of study. Let us stipulate that in a one year study, the risk of relapse off antidepressant increases exponentially over time, so that it is rather low initially and quite high at months 11 and 12. Since this risk of relapse is not a constant slope, it would violate the proportionality assumption, and thus estimates of relative risk compared to another group on antidepressants would not be fully accurate. This problem can be addressed statistically by the use of "time-varying covariate" analyses.

Another problem in Cox regression, less amenable to statistical correction, is the assumption that "censored persons have had the same course (as if they had not been censored) as persons who were not censored. In other words, the losses occur *randomly*, independent of outcome." (Katz, 2003; my italic.) In survival analysis, we are measuring time to an event. The rationale is that in a prospective study, let us say with one-year follow-up, we need to account not only for the frequency of events (how many people relapsed in two arms of a study) but the duration that patients stayed well until the event occurred. Thus, suppose two arms involved treatment with antipsychotics and 50% relapsed in each arm by one year; however in one arm, all 50% had relapsed in the first month of follow-up, while in the second arm, no one relapsed at all for 6 months, and all the other 50% relapsed in the second half of the year. Obviously, the second arm was more effective, delaying time to a relapse. In survival analysis, those patients who stop the study – either because they relapse before the one-year endpoint, or because they have side effects or for whatever reason – are included in the analysis until the time they stop the study. Suppose someone stops the antipsychotic at 3 months, and another person at 9 months, then the data of each person would be included in the analysis until 3 or 9 months, respectively, with the patient being "censored" at that 3 or 9 month time frame, that is, removed from the analysis. The assumption here is that, at the time of censoring, the one patient left the study *randomly* at 3 months, and the other patient stayed in and then left the study *randomly* at 9 months. If there was a systematic bias in the study, some special reason why patients in one arm stayed in the study longer and others did not (like, for example, if one group received an effective study drug and the other did not), then this random censoring assumption would not hold. Or suppose one group non-randomly had more dropouts due to side effects, again the assumption would be broken.

Survival analysis and sample size

In survival analysis, one always needs to know the sample size at each time point; if there are many dropouts, the survival curve may be misleading. Sample size decreases with time in a survival analysis. This is normal and expected, and happens for two reasons: either the endpoint of the study is reached (such as a mood episode relapse), or the patient never experiences the endpoint (either staying well until the end of the study or dropping out of the study for some other reason except the endpoint). Thus, in general, a survival analysis is more valid (because it contains a larger sample) in the earlier parts of the curve, rather than the later parts of the curve. For example, a study may seem to have a major effect after 6 months, but the sample at that point could be 10 patients in each arm, as opposed to 100 patients in each arm at 1 month. The results would not be statistically significant and the effect size would not be meaningful because of the high variability of such small numbers. But to the naked eye, there may seem to be more of an effect than one is justified in accepting. Although this is frequently not done, this problem can be minimized by providing the actual sample size at each month on the survival curve under the x-axis, thus allowing readers to put less weight into apparent differences when the sample size is small. (Conversely, the lack of a difference when sample sizes are small is also unreliable, and thus one should not confidently conclude in that case that there is no effect.)

The problem of dropouts

Survival analysis assumes random dropouts. We know that dropouts are usually not random. So how can we continue to rely on survival analysis? Mainly because we have no other options at this time. Again this highlights the need for recognition of the statistical issues involved, but also for a good deal of caution and humility in interpreting the results of even the best randomized clinical trials. The main statistical issue is that since dropouts are unavoidably non-random, a survival analysis is more valid if there are few dropouts that are due to *loss to follow-up*. What this means is that we really have no idea why the patient has left the study. Statisticians have tended to assign a ballpark figure of 20% loss to follow-up as tolerable over-all so as to maintain reasonable confidence in the validity of a survival analysis. Sometimes a sensitivity analysis can be done, where one assumes a best case scenario (all dropouts remain well) and a worst case scenario (all dropouts relapse) in order to see if the conclusions change. But nonetheless, a high percentage of dropouts means we cannot be certain if our results are valid. In fact, the dropout rates in maintenance studies of bipolar disorder tend to be in the 50% to 80% range, which hampers our ability to be certain of the validity of survival analysis in bipolar research. We must resign ourselves to the fact that this population is difficult to study, interpreting data with caution while rejecting ivory-tower statisticians' rejection of such research.

Residual confounding

All regression models have one final assumption: they "all assume that observations are independent of one another. In other words, these models cannot incorporate the same outcome occurring more than once in the same person." (Katz, 2003.) Thus, if in a one year follow-up, one is measuring the outcome of subsyndromal depressive worsening, and patients go back and forth between being completely asymptomatic and then subsyndromally symptomatic, then they are having the outcome multiple times during follow-up. In this circumstance, one must statistically "adjust for the correlation between repeated observations in the same patients" using "generalized estimating equations." (Katz, 2003.)

No matter how much statistical adjustment is made with regression models, even when all the above assumptions are met, we are always faced with the fact that one can never completely identify and correct for all possible confounding variables. Only a randomized study can approximate that ideal state. Thus, in even the best regression model, there will be *residual confounding*, a left over amount of confounding bias that cannot be completely removed. Although one cannot attain absolute certainty in this regard, one can at least quantify the likely amount of residual confounding, and, if it is rather low, one can be more certain of the results of the regression analysis. (Recall the profound saying of Laplace that the genius of statistics lies in quantifying, rather than ignoring, error.) Residual analysis examines "the differences between the observed and estimated values" (Katz, 2003) in a model; it is a quantification of the "error in estimation." If residual estimations are large, then the model does not fit the data well, either because of failure of some of the assumptions above, or, more commonly, failure in identifying and analyzing important confounding and predictive variables.

Methods of selecting variables for regression models: how to conduct analyses

Perhaps more important even than the above assumptions, researchers who conduct regression analyses have to select variables for their analyses. This is not a simple process, and published studies rarely describe the specifics about how these analyses are conducted, nor, in the interests of practicality, can they do so. Sometimes, to be more transparent, researchers utilize computerized selection models, but these too have their own limitations.

The key issue is that regression models are useless if they do not contain the needed information on confounding variables. Also, in trying to model all the predictors of an outcome, one would want information on other predictors, besides the experimental predictor of interest.

How does one know which variables are confounding factors? How does one know what other variables are predictors of the outcome?

Let us begin with some simple concepts. One should not generally conduct regression analyses in complete ignorance of the previous literature (except, perhaps, in the rare circumstances where a topic has never been studied at all previously). Thus, one should begin with inclusion of variables that other studies have already identified as being potential predictors of an outcome. Even if limited research is available, one can turn to clinical experience (one's own, or common standards of opinion) to identify potential predictive variables. This is totally legitimate and does not imply that one accepts the clinical opinions of others nor that one accepts the prior literature at face value; one will *test* those opinions and previous studies once again in one's own regression analysis. One might even include variables that have never been studied, with purely theoretical justification. Again, this is the first, not the last, step; and it is better to be overinclusive and then remove variables that turn out to have no appreciable impact, rather than to be too picky up front, leaving out variables that are important, and thereby making the model less able to fit the data.

So one begins with variables already suggested by previous research, by clinical experience, and by theoretical rationales. Besides these three starting points, all of which are conceptual, there is one other conceptual starting point that I think is insufficiently appreciated in medical research: social and economic factors. A new literature on social epidemiology is teaching us that social factors, ones that relate to one's class and economic status and race, influence medical outcomes often independent of one's individual features. Usually, much detail on such factors is not available in medical research studies; it is important to start collecting such data, but in lieu of such efforts, a simple observation is relevant: such factors correlate well with some simple demographic features, particularly race, level of education, and where one lives (sometimes assessed by zip code). Age and gender are also important social factors in medical outcomes. Thus, I would suggest that almost all regression models should include race, level of education, age, and gender in their analyses – these serve as proxies for social and economic influences on health and illness.

The handmade method

After these four conceptual factors in choosing variables for a regression model (previous research, clinical experience, theoretical rationales, and social/economic factors), one can then begin a quantitative examination of which variables to include in a model. I will call this process *handmade selection* to distinguish it from computerized selection procedures. (The analogy is to handmade, as opposed to the machine-made, products, like Persian rugs; machines do not always improve upon human protoplasm.)

In handmade selection, the process is roughly as follows: Suppose we have 20 variables on which we have collected data in an observational (non-randomized) study of 100 subjects. The outcome is treatment response (defined as greater than 50% response on a depression rating scale), and thus this dichotomous outcome identifies our model as logistic regression. The main experimental predictor is antidepressant use (let us say one-half of our sample took antidepressants, and the other half did not). We have ten other variables: age, race, gender, number of hospitalizations, number of suicide attempts, past substance abuse, past psychosis, and so on. We then would first put just antidepressant use (let's call it "AD") in the model as the predictor, with treatment response ("TR") as the outcome. The regression model would thus be:

1. TR = AD

This would be simple univariate statistics, or the result of simply comparing AD in those with and without TR. It does not yet take advantage of the benefits of regression. Let's say that this univariate model shows that AD is much higher in treatment responders; this would be seen in an odds ratio (OR) that is large, say 3.50, with confidence intervals (CIs) that do not cross the null (null = 1); let's say that the 95% CIs are 1.48 on the lower end and 8.63 on the higher end. Now we can start adding each variable one by one, choosing whichever we think is most relevant. It might go as follows in successive order of modeling:

2. TR = AD + race
3. TR = AD + race + gender
4. TR = AD + race + gender + number of hospitalizations, and so on.

An example of confounding effects might be noticed in the following scenario: remember the original OR of 3.50 for AD in the univariate comparison. Suppose the OR for AD changed as follows:

2. OR is 2.75 for TR = AD + race
3. OR is 2.70 for TR = AD + race + gender
4. OR is 1.20 for TR = AD + race + gender + number of hospitalizations.

Using the standard criterion of a 10% change in effect size as reflective of confounding bias, we should note that 10% of 3.50 is 0.35. So any change in the effect size of the AD predictor here that is larger than 0.35 should be considered as a possible confounder; larger changes would be seen as more likely to reflect confounding bias. So, in the second step, we see about a 20% decrease in the effect size when race was added. This is common, but the overall effect still seems present, though slightly smaller than it initially seemed. Next, in step 3, we see no notable change when gender was added. Then in step 4, we note a major change in the effect size, becoming almost half in size and approximating the null value of 1.0. If the CIs in step 4 cross the null (let's say they were 0.80 to 1.96), then we could say that no real effect of AD would remain. This example shows how an apparent effect (OR = 3.50 in univariate analysis) may reflect confounding bias (disappear after multivariate regression). Further, one can make sense of the regression findings by noting that adjustment for number of hospitalizations corrects for severity of illness; these results would then suggest that perhaps those who received antidepressants were less severely ill than those who did not receive antidepressants; thus the apparent association of AD with TR was really a simple difference in baseline severity of illness between the two groups. Standard statistics like p-values employed without regression modeling would not correct for this kind of important clinical variable.

The kitchen sink method

Another way to conduct this kind of multivariate regression model is to simply use all those relevant variables all at once, rather than putting them in the model one by one as described above. This alternative approach, sometimes called "the kitchen sink" method, has the benefit of being quick and easy; it has the disadvantage, though, of decreasing the statistical power of the analysis (due to "collinearity": the more variables included in a model, the wider the CIs). Also, it does not allow one to see which specific variables seemed to have the most impact on confounding effects. This latter issue could be addressed by taking each variable out one by one until one sees a major change in the effect size of the experimental variable (like the OR for AD in the example above).

Computerized methods

Some researchers do not like the idea of having to trust other researchers as to how they conduct their regression analyses. One has to go on trust with these handmade methods that researchers are reporting their results honestly and objectively. Suppose, in the above example, that I really believed that antidepressants were effective in that study; suppose further that I conducted the sequential regression model above, and when I got to the fourth step, I became unhappy. I could not accept that antidepressants were ineffective, as a result of confounding bias due to number of past hospitalizations. Let us suppose, then, that I acted dishonestly: I chose to write up the paper with only the first three steps of the regression, not reporting the fourth one. Peer reviewers might or might not ask about severity of illness as a potential confounding factor, but they would not actually be analyzing the data themselves, so no one could check on me to make certain that I conducted the analysis properly.

Now this kind of dishonesty is dangerous, obviously, because it is scientific misconduct. However, one need not posit dishonesty; hand-conducted regression analyses are just difficult to duplicate, just as a handwoven rug is one of a kind. Thus, some researchers prefer computer-conducted regression models, which are at least duplicable in theory, and in which human intervention is absent, for better or worse.

These are the kinds of models one often sees in research papers termed "stepwise conditional regression" or similar terms. Though various types exist, I will simplify to two basic options: forward or backward. The term "conditional" means that each step in the regression is dependent on the previous step.

Forward selection would proceed as in the example above, with each variable added one at a time. However, unlike our handmade model, one has to give the computer a clear and simple rationale for keeping or not keeping a variable. The usual rationale given is a p-value cutoff, frequently 0.05, and sometimes higher (such as 0.10–0.20) to account for the fact that regression models are exploring hypotheses (and thus higher p-values are acceptable) rather than trying to prove hypotheses (where lower p-values are generally accepted). So, in the above example, if gender in step 3 has a p-value of 0.38, it will not be included in step 4.

Backward deletion, which I prefer, begins with the kitchen sink model (including all variables) and then removes them one by one, starting with the highest p-value and going downwards until all remaining variables are lower than the accepted p-value threshold.

These computerized models have the advantage of duplication, but they have the disadvantage of being single-focused: p-values are their sole criterion. They do not assess changes in the experimental effect size (e.g., the OR for AD in the example), and thus they may take out a variable that has a confounding effect (changes in the OR of AD) while not itself being a predictor (its own p-value is high). Thus, in the example above, in step 2, we saw that race was a confounding factor; it changed the OR of AD. Let's say that race itself was not a predictor (its $p = 0.43$); this makes sense because race, by itself, likely does not cause depression as an illness to be more or less severe. This confounding, but not predictor, effect would not be captured by computerized models.

I still prefer the handmade approach to regression, with the proviso that such methods require maximum objectivity and honesty on the part of researchers. For those who mistrust human nature too much for this proposal, the computerized backward conditional approach may be the next best alternative.

References

Abramson, J. (2004) *Ovedosed America: The Broken Promise of American Medicine*. New York: Harper Collins.

Abramson, J. H. and Abramson, Z. H. (2001) *Making Sense of Data: A Self-Instruction Manual on the Interpretation of Epidemiological Data*. New York: Oxford University Press.

Altshuler, L., Suppes, T., Black, D., *et al.* (2003) Impact of antidepressant discontinuation after acute bipolar depression remission on rates of depressive relapse at 1-year follow-up. *Am J Psychiatry*, **160**, 1252–62.

American College of Neuropsychopharmacology (2004) Executive summary: Preliminary report of the task force on SSRI's and suicidal behavior in youth. Available at: www.acnp.org, accessed January 22, 2009.

Andrews, G., Anstey, K., Brodaty, H., Issakidis, C. and Luscombe, G. (1999) Recall of depressive episode 25 years previously. *Psychol Med*, **29**, 787–91.

Angell, M. (2005) *The Truth About the Drug Companies*. New York: Random House.

Barbui, C., Cipriani, A., Malvini, L. and Tansella, M. (2006) Validity of the impact factor of journals as a measure of randomized controlled trial quality. *J Clin Psychiatry*, **67**, 37–40.

Basoglu, M., Marks, I., Livanou, M. and Swinson, R. (1997) Double-blindness procedures, rater blindness, and ratings of outcome. Observations from a controlled trial. *Arch Gen Psychiatry*, **54**, 744–8.

Baxt, W. G., Waeckerle, J. F., Berlin, J. A. and Callaham, M. L. (1998) Who reviews the reviewers? Feasibility of using a fictitious manuscript to evaluate peer reviewer performance. *Ann Emerg Med*, **32**, 310–7.

Bayes, T. and Price, R. (1763) An essay toward solving a problem in the doctrine of chances. *Philos Trans R Soc London*, **53**, 370–418. Available at http://www.stat.ucla.edu/history/essay.pdf.

Benson, K. and Hartz, A. J. (2000) A comparison of observational studies and randomized, controlled trials. *N Engl J Med*, **342**, 1878–86.

Berry, D. A. (1993) A case for Bayesianism in clinical trials. *Stat Med*, **12**, 1377–93; discussion 1395–404.

Blackwelder, W. C. (1982) "Proving the null hypothesis" in clinical trials. *Control Clin Trials*, **3**, 345–53.

Blank, A. (2006) Swan's way. *JAMA*, **296**, 1041–2.

Bolwig, T. G. (2006) Psychiatry and the humanities. *Acta Psychiatr Scand*, **114**, 381–3.

Bowden, C., Calabrese, J., McElroy, S., *et al.* (2000) A randomized, placebo-controlled 12-month trial of divalproex and lithium in treatment of outpatients with bipolar I disorder. *Arch Gen Psychiatry*, **57**, 481–9.

Bowden, C., Calabrese, J., Sachs, G., *et al.* (2003) A placebo-controlled 18-month trial of lamotrigine and lithium maintenance treatment in recently manic or hypomanic patients with bipolar I disorder. *Arch Gen Psychiatry*, **60**, 392–400.

Brown, H. (2007) How impact factors changed medical publishing – and science. *BMJ*, **334**, 561–4.

Buchkowsky, S. S. and Jewesson, P. J. (2004) Industry sponsorship and authorship of clinical trials over 20 years. *Ann Pharmacother*, **38**, 579–85.

Cade, J. F. (1971) Contemporary challenges in psychiatry. *Aust N Z J Psychiatry*, **5**, 10–17.

Calabrese, J. R., Bowden, C. L., Sachs, G. S., *et al.* (1999) A double-blind placebo-controlled study of lamotrigine monotherapy in outpatients with bipolar I depression. Lamictal 602 Study Group. *J Clin Psychiatry*, **60**, 79–88.

Calabrese, J. R., Suppes, T., Bowden, C. L. *et al.* (2000) A double-blind, placebo-controlled, prophylaxis study of lamotrigine in rapid-cycling bipolar disorder. Lamictal 614 Study Group. *J Clin Psychiatry*, **61**, 841–50.

Calabrese, J., Bowden, C., Sachs, G., *et al.* (2003) A placebo-controlled 18-month trial of lamotrigine and lithium maintenance treatment in recently depressed patients with bipolar I disorder. *J Clin Psychiatry*, **64**, 1013–24.

Calabrese, J. R., Keck, P. E., JR., Macfadden, W., *et al.* (2005) A randomized, double-blind, placebo-controlled trial of quetiapine in the treatment of bipolar I or II depression. *Am J Psychiatry*, **162**, 1351–60.

Calabrese, J. R., Huffman, R. F., White, R. L., *et al.* (2008) Lamotrigine in the acute treatment of bipolar depression: results of five double-blind, placebo-controlled clinical trials. *Bipolar Disord*, **10**, 323–33.

Carroll, B. J. (2004) Adolescents with depression. *JAMA*, **292**, 2578.

Carroll, B. J. (2006) Ten rules of academic life: reflections on the career of an affective disorders researcher. *J Affect Disord*, **92**, 7–12.

Cohen, J. (1994) The earth is round (*p* < .05). *Am Psychol*, **49**, 997–1003.

Cohn, J. B., Collins, G., Ashbrook, E. and Wernick, J. F. (1989) A comparison of fluoxetine, imipramine and placebo in patients with bipolar depressive disorder. *Int Clin Psychopharmacol*, **4**, 313–14.

Das, A. K., Olfson, M., Gameroff, M. J., *et al.* (2005) Screening for bipolar disorder in a primary care practice. *JAMA*, **293**, 956–63.

Davidoff, F., Deangelis, C. D., Drazen, J. M., *et al.* (2001) Sponsorship, authorship, and accountability. *JAMA*, **286**, 1232–4.

Dawson, B. and Trapp, R. (2001) *Basic and Clinical Biostatistics*. New York: McGraw-Hill.

Dennett, D. (2000) Postmodernism and truth. In J. Hintikka, S. Neville, E. Sosa and A. Olsen, eds., *Proceedings of the 20th World Congress of Philosophy, Volume 8*. Charlottesville, VA: Philosophy Documentation Center.

Doll, R. (2002) Proof of causality: deduction from epidemiological observation. *Perspect Biol Med*, **45**, 499–515.

Emanuel, E. J. and Miller, F. G. (2001) The ethics of placebo-controlled trials – a middle ground. *N Engl J Med*, **345**, 915–19.

Eysenck, H. J. (1994) Meta-analysis and its problems. *BMJ*, **309**, 789–92.

Feinstein, A. R. (1977) *Clinical Biostatistics*. St. Louis: Mosby.

Feinstein, A. R. (1995) Meta-analysis: statistical alchemy for the 21st century. *J Clin Epidemiol*, **48**, 71–9.

Feinstein, A. R. and Horwitz, R. I. (1997) Problems in the "evidence" of "evidence-based medicine". *Am J Med*, **103**, 529–35.

Fink, M. and Taylor, M. A. (2007) Electroconvulsive therapy: evidence and challenges. *JAMA*, **298**, 330–2.

Fink, M. and Taylor, M. A. (2008) The medical evidence-based model for psychiatric syndromes: return to a classical paradigm. *Acta Psychiatr Scand*, **117**, 81–4.

Fisher, R. (1971 [1935]) *The Design of Experiments*, 9th edn. New York: Macmillan.

Fletcher, W. (1907) Rice and beri-beri: preliminary report on an experiment conducted at the Kuala Lumpur Lunatic Asylum. *Lancet*, **i**, 1776–9.

Forster, E. F. (1979) Some ethical considerations in the development of psychopharmacological research and practice in the future. *Prog Neuropsychopharmacol*, **3**, 277–80.

Foucault, M. (1994) *The Birth of the Clinic*. New York: Vintage.

Friedman, L., Furberg, C. and Demets, D. (1998) *Fundamentals of Clinical Trials*, 3rd edn. New York: Springer.

Gehlbach, S. (2006) *Interpreting the Medical Literature*. New York: McGraw-Hill.

Ghaemi, S. N. (2003) *The Concepts of Psychiatry: A Pluralistic Approach to the Mind and Mental Illness*. Baltimore, MD: Johns Hopkins University Press.

Ghaemi, S. N. (2007) *Mood Disorders: A Practical Guide*, 2nd edn. Philadelphia: Lippincott, Williams, and Wilkins.

Ghaemi, S. N. (2008) Toward a Hippocratic psychopharmacology. *Can J Psychiatry*, **53**, 189–96.

Ghaemi, S. N. and Goodwin, F. K. (2007) The ethics of clinical innovation in psychopharmacology: challenging traditional bioethics. *Philos Ethics Humanit Med*, **2**, 26.

Ghaemi, S. N., Soldani, F. and Hsu, D. J. (2003) Evidence-based pharmacotherapy of bipolar disorder. *Int J Neuropsychopharmacol*, **6**, 303–8.

Ghaemi, S. N., Miller, C. J., Rosenquist, K. J. and Pies, R. (2005) Sensitivity and specificity of the Bipolar Spectrum Diagnostic Scale for detecting bipolar disorder. *J Affect Disord*, **84**, 273–7.

Ghaemi, S. N., Gilmer, W. S., Goldberg, J. F., *et al.* (2007) Divalproex in the treatment of acute bipolar depression: a preliminary double-blind, randomized, placebo-controlled pilot study. *J Clin Psychiatry*, **68**, 1840–4.

Ghaemi, S. N., Shirzadi, A. and Filkowski, M. (2008a) Publication bias and the pharmaceutical industry: the case of lamotrigine in bipolar disorder. *Medscape J Med*, **9**, 211.

Ghaemi, S. N., Wingo, A. P., Filkowski, M. A. and Baldessarini, R. J. (2008b) Long-term antidepressant treatment in bipolar disorder: meta-analyses of benefits and risks. *Acta Psychiatr Scand*, **118**, 347–56.

Gijsman, H. J., Geddes, J. R., Rendell, J. M., Nolen, W. A. and Goodwin, G. M. (2004) Antidepressants for bipolar depression: a systematic review of randomized, controlled trials. *Am J Psychiatry*, **161**, 1537–47.

Goldberg, J. F. and Whiteside, J. E. (2002) The association between substance abuse and antidepressant-induced mania in bipolar disorder: a preliminary study. *J Clin Psychiatry*, **63**, 791–5.

Goodman, S. N. (1999) Toward evidence-based medical statistics. 2: The Bayes factor. *Ann Intern Med*, **130**, 1005–13.

Goodwin, F. K. and Jamison, K. R. (2007) *Manic Depressive Illness*, 2nd edn. New York: Oxford University Press.

Goodwin, G. M., Bowden, C. L., Calabrese, J. R., *et al.* (2004) A pooled analysis of 2 placebo-controlled 18-month trials of lamotrigine and lithium maintenance in bipolar I disorder. *J Clin Psychiatry*, **65**, 432–41.

Gyulai, L., Bowden, C., McElroy, S., *et al.* (2003) Maintenance efficacy of divalproex in the prevention of bipolar depression. *Neuropsychopharmacology*, **28**, 1374–82.

Hammad, T. A., Laughren, T. and Racoosin, J. (2006) Suicidality in pediatric patients treated with antidepressant drugs. *Arch Gen Psychiatry*, **63**, 332–9.

Healy, D. (2001) *The Creation of Psychopharmacology*. Cambridge, MA: Harvard University Press.

Healy, D. (2008) *Mania*. Baltimore: Johns Hopkins University Press.

Hill, A. B. (1962) *Statistical Methods in Clinical and Preventive Medicine*. New York: Oxford University Press.

Hill, A. B. (1965) The environment and disease: association or causation? *Proc R Soc Med*, **58**, 295–300.

Hill, A. B. (1971) *Principles of Medical Statistics*, 9th edn. New York: Oxford University Press.

Hirschfeld, R. M., Williams, J. B., Spitzer, R. L., *et al.* (2000) Development and validation of a screening instrument for bipolar spectrum disorder: the Mood Disorder Questionnaire. *Am J Psychiatry*, **157**, 1873–5.

Hirschfeld, R. M., Calabrese, J. R., Weissman, M. M., *et al.* (2003) Screening for bipolar disorder in the community. *J Clin Psychiatry*, **64**, 53–9.

Horton, R. (2002a) The hidden research paper. *JAMA*, **287**, 2775–8.

Horton, R. (2002b) Postpublication criticism and the shaping of clinical knowledge. *JAMA*, **287**, 2843–7.

Horton, R. (2004) The dawn of McScience. *New York Review of Books*, **51**, 7–9.

Hrobjartsson, A. and Gotzsche, P. C. (2001) Is the placebo powerless? An analysis of clinical trials comparing placebo with no treatment. *N Engl J Med*, **344**, 1594–602.

Hummer, M., Holzmeister, R., Kemmler, G., *et al.* (2003) Attitudes of patients with schizophrenia toward placebo-controlled clinical trials. *J Clin Psychiatry*, **64**, 277–81.

Hunt, M. (1997) *How Science Takes Stock: The Story of Meta-Analysis*. London: Russell Sage Foundation.

Ioannidis, J. P. (2005) Contradicted and initially stronger effects in highly cited clinical research. *JAMA*, **294**, 218–28.

Jaeschke, R., Guyatt, G. and Sackett, D. L. (1994) Users' guides to the medical literature. III. How to use an article about a diagnostic test. A. Are the results of the study valid? Evidence-Based Medicine Working Group. *JAMA*, **271**, 389–91.

James, W. (1956 [1897]) Is life worth living? *The Will to Believe and Other Essays in Popular Philosophy*. New York: Dover.

Jaspers, K. (1997 [1959]) *General Psychopathology: Volumes 1 and 2*. Baltimore, MD: Johns Hopkins University Press.

Jefferson, T., Alderson, P., Wager, E. and Davidoff, F. (2002) Effects of editorial peer review: a systematic review. *JAMA*, **287**, 2784–6.

Joffe, R. T., MacQueen, G. M., Marriott, M. and Young, L. T. (2005) One-year outcome with antidepressant–treatment of bipolar depression. *Acta Psychiatr Scand*, **112**, 105–9.

Jorge, R. E., Robinson, R. G., Arndt, S. and Starkstein, S. (2003) Mortality and poststroke depression: a placebo-controlled trial of antidepressants. *Am J Psychiatry*, **160**, 1823–9.

Kanigel, R. (1986) *Apprentice to Genius: The Making of a Scientific Dynasty*. New York: Macmillan.

Katz, M. (2003) Multivariable analysis: a primer for readers of medical research. *Ann Intern Med*, **138**, 644–50.

Keitner, G. I., Solomon, D. A., Ryan, C. E., *et al.* (1996) Prodromal and residual symptoms in bipolar I disorder. *Compr Psychiatry*, **37**, 362–7.

Kennedy, J. (1962) *Public Papers of the Presidents of the United States*. Washington DC: Office of the Federal Register.

Kent, D. M. and Hayward, R. A. (2007) Limitations of applying summary results of clinical trials to individual patients: the need for risk stratification. *JAMA*, **298**(10), 1209–12.

Kirsch, I., Deacon, B. J., Huedo-medina, T. B., *et al.* (2008) Initial severity and antidepressant benefits: a meta-analysis of data submitted to the Food and Drug Administration. *PLoS Med*, **5**, e45.

Kojeve, A. (1980) *Introduction to the Reading of Hegel*. New York: Cornell University Press.

Kraemer, H. C. and Kupfer, D. J. (2006) Size of treatment effects and their importance to clinical research and practice. *Biol Psychiatry*, **59**, 990–6.

Kushner, S. F., Khan, A., Lane, R. and Olson, W. H. (2006) Topiramate monotherapy in the management of acute mania: results of four double-blind placebo-controlled trials. *Bipolar Disord*, **8**, 15–27.

Lang, J. M., Rothman, K. J. and Cann, C. I. (1998) That confounded P-value. *Epidemiology*, **9**, 7–8.

Leon, A. C. (2004) Multiplicity-adjusted sample size requirements: a strategy to maintain statistical power with Bonferroni adjustments. *J Clin Psychiatry*, **65**, 1511–4.

Levine, R. and Fink, M. (2006) The case against evidence-based principles in psychiatry. *Med Hypotheses*, **67**, 401–10.

Lexchin, J., Bero, L. A., Djulbegovic, B. and Clark, O. (2003) Pharmaceutical industry sponsorship and research outcome and quality: systematic review. *BMJ*, **326**, 1167–70.

Louis, P. C. A. (1835) Researches on the Effects of Bloodletting in some Inflammatory Diseases. (Reprinted by the Classics of Medicine Library, Birmingham, Alabama, 1986.)

Mack, J. (1995) *Abduction: Human Encounters with Aliens*. New York: Ballantine.

Mackay, A. (1991) *A Dictionary of Scientific Quotations*. Boca Raton, FL: CRC Press.

Makkreel, R. (1992) *Dilthey: Philosopher of the Human Studies*. Princeton, NJ: Princeton University Press.

Manwani, S. G., Pardo, T. B., Albanese, *et al.* (2006) Substance use disorder and other predictors of antidepressant-induced mania: a retrospective chart review. *J Clin Psychiatry*, **67**, 1341–5.

March, J., Silva, S., Petrycki, S., *et al.* (2004) Fluoxetine, cognitive-behavioral therapy, and their combination for adolescents with depression: Treatment for Adolescents With Depression Study (TADS) randomized controlled trial. *JAMA*, **292**, 807–20.

McHugh, P. R. (1996) Hippocrates a la mode. *Nat Med*, **2**, 507–9.

Menand, L. (2001) *The Metaphysical Club*. New York: Farrar, Strauss, and Giroux.

Miettinen, O. and Cook, E. (1981) Confounding: essence and detection. *Am J Epidemiol*, **114**, 593–603.

Miller, C. J., Klugman, J. Berv, D. A., Rasenquist, K. J. and Ghaemi, S. N. (2004) Sensitivity and specificity of the Mood Disorder Questionnaire for detecting bipolar disorder. *J Affect Disord*, **81**, 161–71.

Mills, C. (1963) *Power, Politics, and People*. New York: Oxford University Press.

Moncrieff, J., Wessely, S. and Hardy, R. (1998) Meta-analysis of trials comparing antidepressants with active placebos. *Br J Psychiatry*, **172**, 227–31; discussion 232–4.

Moynihan, R. (2008) Key opinion leaders: independent experts or drug representatives in disguise? *BMJ*, **336**, 1402–3.

Moynihan, R., Heath, I. and Henry, D. (2002) Selling sickness: the pharmaceutical industry and disease mongering. *BMJ*, **324**, 886–91.

National Institute of Health (1979) *The Belmont Report: Ethical Principles and Guidelines for the Protection of Human Subjects of Research*. Washington DC: US Government Printing Office.

Nemeroff, C. B., Evans, D. L., Gyulai, L., *et al.* (2001) Double-blind, placebo-controlled comparison of imipramine and paroxetine in the treatment of bipolar depression. *Am J Psychiatry*, **158**, 906–12.

Olmsted, J. (1952) *Claude Bernard and the Experimental Method in Medicine*. London: H. Schuman.

Osler, W. (1932) *Aequanimitas with other Addresses*. Philadelphia: P. Blakiston's Son and Co.

Pande, A. C., Crockatt, J. G., Janney, C. A., Werth, J. L. and Tsaroucha, G. (2000) Gabapentin in bipolar disorder: a placebo-controlled trial of adjunctive therapy. Gabapentin Bipolar Disorder Study Group. *Bipolar Disord*, **2**, 249–55.

Parascandola, M. (2004) Skepticism, statistical methods, and the cigarette: a historical analysis of a methodological debate. *Perspect Biol Med*, **47**, 244–61.

Parker, G., Tully, L., Olley, A. and Hadzi-Pavlovic, D. (2006) SSRIs as mood stabilizers for Bipolar II Disorder? A proof of concept study. *J Affect Disord*, **92**, 205–14.

Patsopoulos, N. A., Ioannidis, J. P. and Analatos, A. A. (2006) Origin and funding of the most frequently cited papers in medicine: database analysis. *BMJ*, **332**, 1061–4.

Peirce, C. (1958) P. Weiner, Ed., *Selected Writings*. New York: Dover Publications.

Phelps, J. R. and Ghaemi, S. N. (2006) Improving the diagnosis of bipolar disorder: predictive value of screening tests. *J Affect Disord*, **92**, 141–8.

Poe, E. (1845) The system of Dr. Tarr and Prof. Fether. *Graham's Magazine*, Vol XXVIII, No. 5, p. 194.

Pollard, P., & Richardson, J. T. E. (1987) On the probability of making Type I errors. *Psychol Bull*, **102**, 159–163.

Popper, K. (1959) *The Logic of Scientific Discovery*. New York: Basic Books.

Porter, R. (1997) *The Greatest Benefit to Mankind: A Medical History of Humanity*. New York: Norton.

Posternak, M. A. and Zimmerman, M. (2003) How accurate are patients in reporting their antidepressant treatment history? *J Affect Disord*, **75**, 115–24.

Prentice, R. L., Langer, R. D., Stefanick, M. L., *et al.* (2006) Combined analysis of Women's Health Initiative observational and clinical trial data on postmenopausal hormone treatment and cardiovascular disease. *Am J Epidemiol*, **163**, 589–99.

Roberts, L. W., Warner, T. D., Brody, J. L., *et al.* (2002) Patient and psychiatrist ratings of hypothetical schizophrenia research protocols: assessment of harm potential and factors influencing participation decisions. *Am J Psychiatry*, **159**, 573–84.

Robin, E. D. (1985) The cult of the Swan-Ganz catheter. Overuse and abuse of pulmonary flow catheters. *Ann Intern Med*, **103**, 445–9.

Robins, E. and Guze, S. B. (1970) Establishment of diagnostic validity in psychiatric illness: its application to schizophrenia. *Am J Psychiatry*, **126**, 983–7.

Ross, J. S., Hill, K. P., Egilman, D. S. and Krumholz, H. M. (2008) Guest authorship and ghostwriting in publications related to rofecoxib: a case study of industry documents from rofecoxib litigation. *JAMA*, **299**, 1800–12.

Rothman, K. J. and Greenland, S. (1998) *Modern Epidemiology*. Philadelphia: Lippincott-Raven.

Sachs, G. S., Grossman, F., Ghaemi, S. N., Okamoto, A. and Bowden, C. L. (2002) Combination of a mood stabilizer with risperidone or haloperidol for treatment of acute mania: a double-blind, placebo-controlled comparison of efficacy and safety. *Am J Psychiatry*, **159**, 1146–54.

Sachs, G. S., Nierenberg, A. A., Calabrese, J. R., *et al.* (2007) Effectiveness of adjunctive antidepressant treatment for bipolar depression. *N Engl J Med*, **356**, 1711–22.

Sackett, D., Strauss, S., Richardson, W., Rosenberg, W. and Haynes, R. (2000) *Evidence Based Medicine*. London: Churchill Livingstone.

Salsburg, D. (2001) *The Lady Tasting Tea: How Statistics Revolutionized Science in the Twentieth century*. New York: W. H. Freeman and Company.

Shepherd, M. (1993) The placebo: from specificity to the non-specific and back. *Psychol Med*, **23**, 569–78.

Silberman, E. K. and Snyderman, D. A. (1997) Research without external funding in North American psychiatry. *Am J Psychiatry*, **154**, 1159–60.

Silverman, W. (1998) *Where's the Evidence? Debates in Modern Medicine*. New York: Oxford University Press.

Sleight, P. (2000) Debate: subgroup analyses in clinical trials: fun to look at – but don't believe them! *Curr Control Trials Cardiovasc Med*, **1**, 25–7.

Smith, G. and Pell, J. (2003) Parachute use to prevent death and major trauma related to gravitational challenge: systematic review of randomized controlled trials. *BMJ*, **327**, 1459–61.

Soldani, F., Ghaemi, S. N. and Baldessarini, R. (2005) Research methods in psychiatric treatment studies. Critique and proposals. *Acta Psychiatr Scand*, **112**, 1–3.

Sonis, J. (2004) Mortality and poststroke depression. *Am J Psychiatry*, **161**, 1506–7; author reply 1507–8.

Sox, H. C. and Rennie, D. (2006) Research misconduct, retraction, and cleansing the medical literature: lessons from the Poehlman case. *Ann Intern Med*, **144**, 609–13.

Sprock, J. (1988) Classification of schizoaffective disorder. *Compr Psychiatry*, **29**, 55–71.

Stahl, S. M. (2002) Antipsychotic polypharmacy: evidence based or eminence based? *Acta Psychiatr Scand*, **106**, 321–2.

Stahl, S. M. (2005) *Essential Psychopharmacology*. Cambridge, UK: Cambridge University Press.

Stigler, S. (1986) *The History of Statistics: The Measurement of Uncertainty Before 1900*. Cambridge, MA: Harvard University Press.

Tatsioni, A., Bonitsis, N. G. and Ioannidis, J. P. (2007) Persistence of contradicted claims in the literature. *JAMA*, **298**, 2517–26.

Tohen, M., Vieta, E., Calabrese, J., *et al.* (2003) Efficacy of olanzapine and olanzapine-fluoxetine combination in the treatment of bipolar I depression. *Arch Gen Psychiatry*, **60**, 1079–88.

Tohen, M., Chengappa, K. N., Suppes, T., *et al.* (2004) Relapse prevention in bipolar I disorder: 18-month comparison of olanzapine plus mood stabiliser v. mood stabiliser alone. *Br J Psychiatry*, **184**, 337–45.

Turner, E. H., Matthews, A. M., Linardatos, E., Tell, R. A. and Rosenthal, R. (2008) Selective publication of antidepressant trials and its influence on apparent efficacy. *N Engl J Med*, **358**, 252–60.

Wang, R., Lagakos, S. W., Ware, J. H., Hunter, D. J. and Drazen, J. M. (2007) Statistics in medicine–reporting of subgroup analyses in clinical trials. *N Engl J Med*, **357**, 2189–94.

Yastrubetskaya, O., Chiu, E. and O'Connell, S. (1997) Is good clinical research practice for clinical trials good clinical practice? *Int J Geriatr Psychiatry*, **12**, 227–31.

Zimmerman, M., Mattia, J. I. and Posternak, M. A. (2002) Are subjects in pharmacological treatment trials of depression representative of patients in routine clinical practice? *Am J Psychiatry*, **159**, 469–73.

Index

Note: page numbers in *italics* refer to figures and tables